Recovery with Aphasia

University of Illinois Press *Urbana Chicago London*

C. SCOTT MOSS

Recovery with Aphasia

THE AFTERMATH OF MY STROKE

© 1972 by The Board of Trustees
of the University of Illinois
Manufactured in the United States of America
Library of Congress Catalog Card No. 72-074140
ISBN 0-252-00271-7

In memory of my mother

Preface

What began as a short journal article on my tussle with aphasia lengthened into a monograph-sized treatise and finally into this book, describing how my wife and I, and to some extent our children, friends, and associates, reacted to my having sustained a near-fatal stroke; our frantic searching for professional guidance; and what we finally did through repeated trials to combat the thought and language disabilities.

The account is subjectively accurate, since I began dictating notes as soon as I was able, which meant three and a half months after the stroke, and we expanded upon them periodically from that date forward. Writing this manuscript became an obsession with me actually, largely because of the reasons outlined in Chapter 3, but even more, because we began to have indications that we could surmount my overt or public difficulties to a large degree.

Both my wife and I have written not too gently about our initial frustrations, a fact which reflects, of course, the great emotional tension we were under; but in trying to capture exactly what it was like, we also hope that it serves to remind the community that the person who suffers extensive cerebral damage — like the victim of any other major assault — needs greater assistance than is presently available. If one can generalize from my case, early help can indeed be beneficial.

We feel fortunate to have gotten through the ordeal only so slightly scathed. Because of my profession, we had the best medical, psychiatric, and psychological help available, including speech therapy, hypnotherapy, and behavior modification. I doubtlessly profited from each of these (although in each instance I had to reconcile the specific treatment with the personal values I had gleaned from two decades of psychological services).

The major part of this book deals with the lengthy and somewhat tiresome process of rehabilitation and the trial-and-error efforts at self-help that we were forced to devise. Most of it is a testimonial to the love and creativity, the persistence and downright perseverance of my wife, without whose devotion I am absolutely convinced this manuscript could not have been written.

In addition, I would like to single out the assistance of Professor William Brewer, an authority on psycholinguistics, who carefully went over the entire manuscript and gave many thoughtful reactions, and two devoted secretaries, Ann Voss and Mary Jo Fizer.

C. Scott Moss
Santa Ynez, California
1972

Contents

1

The Accident and
the Ensuing Six Months

In September, 1967, I left a position as mental health consultant for the National Institute of Mental Health in San Francisco, where I had enjoyed six years of productive service in promoting the National Mental Health Program in the western region of the U.S. Public Health Service, and took a job as professor of clinical psychology at the University of Illinois. I was returning to the university where I had originally taken my graduate training, and I considered it a distinct honor to be invited back to teach at my alma mater. I was slated to initiate a program in community mental health. The move back to the Midwest did not proceed too smoothly, however; my son Joel fell and broke his arm on the first day of school while we were still in San Carlos. He required surgery and it was decided that the family should remain while I went on ahead.

I lodged in the apartment of my mother, who had preceded us from San Carlos. She had dumped her many cartons into an apartment and departed for Madison, Wisconsin, our original home. I was thankful that at least I had a bed on which to sleep. In the first week of October, I took a flight back to San Francisco, my family met me at the airport with the car fully loaded, and we began immediately the long drive back to Urbana. I had already found a house to rent and shortly thereafter the moving van appeared with the furniture. In the next week we got both the Moss households settled.

The week following I departed for a symposium on the "New Biology of Dreaming" at the University of Cincinnati Medical School. It was a very cold day and the train from Champaign to Chicago had no heat. I began to develop what seemed to be a bad cold that continued to plague me for the next two weeks. Of course, during all this time I was undergoing a general orientation to university life, there were courses to prepare, and I was beginning to meet the many demands of my graduate students. Just before departing for Cincinnati, for instance, I gave a large group of graduate students and faculty a colloquium address on the scope of things to come in the nationally developing community mental health program. So while things were hectic, I would say that they were no more so than the usual pace of my professional and personal life for the last twenty years. I had no impending awareness at all of any catastrophe.

On Monday, October 30, I was working in my office at about four o'clock when a colleague of mine, Len Ullmann, came in. It was during this session that I experienced an abrupt coughing spell which I attributed to his cigarette smoke. I excused myself and went to the drinking fountain, and after a few minutes the coughing subsided. However, I noticed then that vision in my right eye had become askewed. Also, the thumb on my right hand had become numb. I attempted to continue working, but my vision prevented concentration on the written material. So at a few minutes before five I decided to go home. I commented to my wife on my peculiar symptoms, but actually regarded them as only minor, though troublesome, afflictions that I hoped would soon pass.

After dinner I again attempted to read the newspaper, but couldn't, and I began to experience a sharp pain that was at first in the back of my head and then moved to the left side of my temple. I have never been bothered by headaches and I suppose this should have alerted me that something was terribly amiss, but it didn't. My wife fixed a hot water bottle and I held it to the side of my head. By about ten o'clock the pain had somewhat subsided though my eyesight had not improved, and I settled down to try to watch a replay of a recent Green Bay–Bears game.

At about eleven o'clock I experienced another coughing spell, and this one would not stop. My wife became frightened and, wishing to believe that I was teasing her, turned off the TV. Despite my coughing I made a move toward the TV, only to find myself on the floor. Though I did not realize it at the time, the right side of my body had become paralyzed. Bette thought for a moment that I was malingering; however, as she explained to me much later, she knew something had happened when I tried to smile at her and only the left side of my face lit up. I heard her go to the phone and summon an ambulance. She then came back beside me and attempted to subdue my further efforts to rise.

I was conscious or at least semiconscious the whole time. I vaguely remember seeing the ambulance drivers coming in, being rolled onto a cot, feeling rain fall on my face, hearing the sound of the distant siren, and being taken to the emergency room at a local hospital. There was a nurse and also an attendant there who tried to speak with me. Things were hazy but I was in no pain, although I could not talk back to them. Eventually my wife arrived, having called the director of the clinical psychology division, Don Peterson, who came and stayed with the children while Bette came to the hospital. At about one o'clock the doctor in charge of the emergency calls arrived. I then did in retrospect an amazing thing: the paralysis had largely left me and I shifted over on my side and proceeded to engage in an appropriate conversation, experiencing only one or two blocks.

I was then wheeled upstairs to the pediatrics ward, since there were no beds on the adult wards. Bette stayed with me until almost three o'clock. For some reason I remember feeling very depressed. One could call it a premonition of things to come. Just that morning I had taken and passed my physical exam for incoming faculty members. Thinking about it months later, it became obvious to me that such examinations are limited in value in the absence of specific symptoms, since a few hours after the exam I was to suffer a debilitating stroke.

The next morning when I awoke, I was completely and totally aphasic. I was given a neurological examination, an EEG, and later a chest X-ray. As I learned later, the hospital simply lacked skilled clinicians to diagnose my case, though obviously I was a severely brain-damaged patient. On the fourth day, at the insistence of my wife, I was transferred by ambulance to Presbyterian–St. Luke's Hospital in Chicago. My wife and my mother accompanied me in the ambulance. For eight days the staff there pried and prodded me: a brain scan, spinal tap, skull films, and an angiogram were among the techniques utilized.

My life as a patient was uneventful. I was still in no pain. For the most part, I simply slept or dozed. I did comprehend somewhat vaguely what was said to me, but I could not answer except in gestures or by neologisms. I knew the language I used was not correct but I was quite unable to select the appropriate words. I recollect trying to read the headlines of the *Chicago Tribune* but they didn't make any sense to me at all. I didn't have any difficulty focusing; it was simply that the words, individually or in combination, didn't have meaning, and even more amazing, I was only a trifle bothered by that fact.

My wife and my mother were with me and they helped comfort me, feeding me at mealtime and keeping me company. My appetite was largely delinquent, and in the next couple of weeks my weight fell twenty pounds. I did not have a bowel movement during the week I was hospitalized, and fortunately or otherwise no one thought to check on it. I did feel critical (and still do) about the way I was handled by the two surgical residents assigned to my case. Quite unintentionally they imparted the feeling that they were only interested in my *neurological* impairment, and didn't respond to me as a whole human being, one filled with *psychological* reactions at having suffered a catastrophic accident. I attributed this initially to the fact that I couldn't communicate with them and therefore was not sensitive to their interactions with me. Now I realize that this was standard procedure for neurosurgeons, but I still think it is a shame not to treat the patient as a whole personality.

As I look back on it now, I had relatively little concern for the children, my wife, or the home — I was too far out of it to care. I had come so very close to death that I more or less welcomed it. It was indeed, as I experienced it, a very painless way to go. In fact, for a long time afterward I was confident that I was living on borrowed time, and I expected it to expire at any moment. It was as if the stroke had benumbed any emotional investment in the future and I simply shrugged at my perception of my imminent demise.

At the end of a full week, and again at the behest of my wife, I was discharged. A student and his wife drove our car to Chicago and I recall that I was slightly chagrined that I could not converse with them on the drive home. A colleague and his wife had stayed at the house with the children and apparently they all got along very well. It was nice to be in familiar surroundings again.

For a month I stayed in bed or lounged about the house in my bathrobe. A few words of halting, limited speech began to come back to me. Eventually it was time to go to the office again. My wife transported me to and from campus for the next three weeks. They were only token visits and I would stay for about half an hour. Later, when I began driving myself, it was at first strange. It was as if I were learning to coordinate the visual-motor function all over again. The members of the staff seemed glad to see me, and it was nice to be back again, but the difference was simply enormous. I was unable to engage in even normal conversation, let alone deal with more elaborate conceptions. For instance, despite my best efforts I would block even on the most minimal words. Holding a minor conversation of even a few words would be quite taxing for me. I could never tell if what I had to say would come out right — even asking for a pencil from the secretary had to be elaborately planned and painfully carried out.

The second week I ran into a colleague who happened to mention that it must be very frustrating for me to be aphasic since prior to that I had been so verbally facile. I assured him that it was not upsetting and then later found myself wondering why it was not. I think part of the explanation was relatively simple. If I had lost the ability to converse with others, I had also lost the ability even to engage in self-talk. In other words, I did not have the ability to think about the future — to worry, to anticipate or perceive it — at least not with words. Thus, for the first five or six weeks after hospitalization I simply existed. So the fact that I could not use words even internally was, in fact, a safeguard. I imagine it was somewhat similar to undergoing a lobotomy or lobectomy in the dissociation from the future. It was as if without words I could not be concerned about tomorrow.

In the period of January 9 to January 23, I had two meetings in Chicago with Dr. Joseph Wepman, a psychological expert in aphasia. Bette accompanied me by train on the 125-mile trip. I was given a series of tests, and while my performance was of a high level compared to the average brain-damaged patient, nevertheless I was aware of some impairment on the items. I had extreme difficulty in following abstractions of a professional nature (I could follow the meaning of a single sentence but I had difficulty in comprehending the whole). Similarly, I had difficulty in following a digit span for more than five or six numbers (less backwards) and also in defining proverbs (I could still define them at an abstract level but now I had to work around to the answer rather than going directly to it as I had done before). I also had decided deficits in memory. Immediately upon my return from Presbyterian–St. Luke's, I sat down with my wife and tried to remember the names of people we had known in San Carlos; while I was able to picture them, I was completely unable to recall their names, even those of our two next-door neighbors.

It was with regard to a summary meeting with Dr. Wepman in about the middle of January that I found myself while in the bathtub actually beginning to anticipate the rudiments of a discussion that I would have with him.[1] Thus, for the first time I was aware that my inner speech was returning. It is difficult to explain what it was like to be entirely without internal verbalizations. I bathed, shaved, and selected my clothing with appropriateness, for instance, on the few occasions when I got dressed, but without words to express what I was doing, even to myself. It was as though I could perform the automatic habits that I had learned through a lifetime, but would be lost once the demands were made for increasing abstractness.

At this meeting on the 23rd, Dr. Wepman reported that I had improved greatly in the three-week interim, and that in several more months I should be largely restored. He did not have knowledge of what had actually happened to me, because he had not had access to the medical report. He assumed that fat had been given off from the heart, had blocked the carotid artery temporarily, and then had been dissolved. He stated that if the block had remained lodged for even four or five minutes, I would have become a "vegetable." He also said I would continue to manifest organic symptoms for the next several months, but he saw no reason to continue seeing me since I would readily improve. He would be happy to see me in the spring when I was recovered! He concluded that since I had absolutely no premorbid signs this was a "one-time" thing for me.

---

[1] I used to love hot baths during this period. I liked to soak for 45 minutes to an hour, two or even three times a day. Lest the psychodynamically inclined be tempted to overinterpret, this was because the house we had rented turned out to be incompletely insulated.

Finally, he stated that I would benefit little from seeing a speech therapist. From his point of view, time was the primary factor in my recovery, and this was a physiological rather a psychological factor. It was in this conversation that he happened to remark that Dr. Erika Fromm (also at the University of Chicago) had worked for the past couple of years with hypnosis in simulating organic symptoms in normal subjects. I at once replied that I knew Erika and it would be interesting to provide her a brain-injured patient, myself, and see what she could do about restoring normality through hypnosis and age regression. Hypnosis and hypnotherapy had been an interest of mine throughout my professional career.

From that date until early in March I continued to improve. I could exchange pleasantries with a person as long as it was not expected that I would initiate topics or provide much information. I still was unable to hande the abstractions involved in clinical work. I could not read literature or really talk with my colleagues about professional issues. My wife and I nevertheless worked as hard as we were able to recapture my facility with professional jargon and to renew my acquaintance with abstract conceptions. Around the time that I began to visit my office again, we sat down to work on five papers which I had committed myself to complete. The first paper was a survey on the "Experimental Induction of Dreams." Fortunately, I had progressed considerably on the paper before my accident, but it still had to be finished, tidied up, and typed.

I cannot begin to describe how immensely difficult it was to read and summarize the various passages that still remained. It was an unholy, tortuous business. I attempted to dictate to Bette what I wanted to say, and not being able to do this, I reacted strongly at times, sometimes pounding my fists or simply repeating the same gibberish over and over. The normal anxiety over my immediate performance was obviously beginning to return. It seemed so much easier to have my wife read the passages and have me somehow, with her great assistance, manage to indicate what should be done with them. I would stumble about, trying somehow to voice the meaning, my wife would listen to me for some period of time, and then attempt to repeat the gist of what I had to say. Often we would go round and round on certain issues. The result was that the paper ended up half mine and half her own translation of what she thought I had meant to convey. The editors' acceptance of the paper a few weeks later greatly buoyed our spirits (Moss, 1968). Gradually, over some months, as I did a better job of dictating, these extremely difficult periods tended to subside, although I have always been critical about my performance without really being able to do much about it.

On February 1 I volunteered to take on a section of eight students, monitoring them in psychotherapy. Don Peterson was delighted, but I did this with considerable hesitance. It was again a matter of my walking a narrow line between what I was able to do and what I could not yet afford to do. I could not speak with the students at all in the way that I formerly had, being unable to discuss the therapy recordings in detail or their ramifications. Nevertheless, I could deal with questions in a sort of nondirective fashion, as long as too copious an answer wasn't demanded. I also listened to the student-client recordings between sessions and directed Bette to transcribe selected responses while trying not to rob the sessions of all their spontaneity in the process. I managed to complete the course in June, and the students were most generous in their ratings of my performance, though I felt much less than adequate.

It was of interest to me how in a day or even an hour I could feel relatively good and the next moment regress. This matter of recovery is an uncertain thing — it is an uphill struggle of a most uneven character. When I responded to external demands, I could marshal unusual effort for a limited time; for example, when talking on the telephone with the friends and acquaintances who called us I was probably at my optimum. It reminded me of having heard of stutterers who lose their speech defect on the phone. It may have had some relationship to the restricted number of stimuli which I was forced to cope with on the phone. But given time to sit around the house and dwell on my symptoms, or in any type of direct interpersonal relationship and every contact extended me, I was immediately reminded of my glaring deficiencies.

I also found that I was easily distracted; for example, I was not too restrained with the children. Before, I had been able to select what I wanted to watch on TV and noises had not bothered me. But now I found that any distraction was quite upsetting, and I reacted by removing the offender or turning up the volume on the TV until the noise became intolerable to others. On the other side, the TV was a great pacifier: I could vicariously enjoy the human interactions without being called upon to participate.

In February, 1968, I began therapy with the university speech department. I felt that there was virtue in giving my wife some respite from my many demands on her. I met twice a week with a young graduate trainee who was unstructured in her demands but who gave me her undivided attention for an hour each week. On February 27 I reported that for the first time since my accident I remembered a dream. It was of interest to me that for the four-month period I did not recall a single dream. This struck me as a curious state of affairs since for years I had been interested in the study and meaning of dreams; however, my stroke apparently impaired either the ability to have dreams or my capacity to remember them. I lay down each night for seven or eight hours of uninterrupted sleep. It was as if during the daytime I had no words to express what was happening and at night I had no dreams — it was a complete and total vacuum of self-speech for me.

Perhaps Greenberg and Dewan (1968) are correct in saying that in aphasia dreaming serves to integrate new information into existing past information stores. I tended to dream in pictures, of course, but without words the memory of these nocturnal images was lost. Since my big white boxer dog "dreams" every evening without words, for example, this leads to the speculation that perhaps I didn't dream during the recovery period from my accident. How else would one account for the fact that even today I hold many waking memories from my period of hospitalization and the first few months when I had no words to describe these events even to myself, but at the same time do not remember having dreamed at all during these four months. Further evidence is that as I recovered my internal verbalizations, the memory of nocturnal mentation began to recur.

When I entered into ordinary conversation after five or six months, I had progressed sufficiently to talk more or less normally until I came to a word on which I might block. Unlike former times at that juncture, *absolutely nothing* came to mind — it was an absolute zero — there were no alternatives from which to choose. I purchased a crossword puzzle book to give me facility in learning synonyms. The problem of dealing with abstractions also continued to plague me during this period. It took a great deal of effort for me to keep an abstraction in mind. For example, in talking with the speech therapist I would begin to give a definition of an abstract concern, but as I held it in mind it would sort of fade, and chances were that I'd end up giving a simplified version rather than one at the original level of conception. It was as though giving an abstraction required so much of my addled intelligence that halfway through the definition I would run out of the energy available to me and regress to a more concrete answer. Something like this happened again and again.

It was also fascinating to me how completely and totally fixed I was on the "here and now." Even former events just prior to my accident had faded. In regard to my professional work, I recognized the terms that were used, but in a sense they had receded into the distant past rather than being immediately in my awareness. And in the same vein, thought about the future was most difficult. So both the past and the future had faded for me, and I existed almost exclusively in the present. In working with my speech therapist, for instance, I had been attempting to explain the general conceptions of community health. As long as I stuck to the paper or an outline, I did relatively well. But without the outline I rapidly floundered, although I could answer specific questions that were asked. In essence, then, I was unable to keep in mind a verbal outline of what I had to say. This in broader perspective is what happened to me generally. I was unable to generate a gestalt of either my previous life or the future, and therefore life beyond the immediate situation was meaningless. This restriction held not only for my work but for all personal life as well. For example, five months after the accident I was able to recall occasionally the names of some people who were our San Carlos neighbors, but I could not embroider them with associations as I had formerly.

From March 14 through March 18 I was a patient at Michael Reese Hospital, where I had volunteered as an experimental subject for Dr. Doris Gruenewald, a colleague of Erika Fromm whom I had also met previously. I traveled to Chicago without my wife, which indicates that I was making some progress. It was Dr. Gruenewald's job, if possible, to induce me into hypnosis, cause me to regress beyond the time when I had suffered my stroke, and determine whether I had recovered, to any appreciable extent, my normal method of speaking and thinking. It was at best a far-out experimental effort which reflected my desperation that hypnotheraphy might help.

I was admitted to a locked psychiatric ward in which most of the patients had partial "open-door privileges." It was a peculiar and unique personal experience for anyone, especially for a clinical psychologist who often had wondered what the experience would be like behind locked doors. I was treated exactly the same as all the other patients; for instance, the nurses immediately went through my suitcase and took my medicine and my razor. Prior to any attempts at hypnosis, I was given a complete physical and neurological examination. I passed the examination in excellent shape. I also had a prehypnotic EEG taken while I was in a drugged sleep. The reason for this phase of the study was a report by Kupper in 1945. Through hypnotic age-regression he had supposedly transported an epileptic patient back beyond the period of traumatic injury and what had previously been very morbid then turned into a normal-appearing electroencephalogram. I was extremely skeptical of this experiment; no one had replicated the study to my knowledge.

During the examination with Doris Gruenewald, it occurred to me to tell her of an experience which I had suffered twenty-two years before. I was stationed for the last year of military service in World War II with a B-29 group on Guam. When we were not busy with the planes, we used to play a great deal of bridge, often three to five hours a day. In the middle of February, 1946, I was transported back to the United States and in a couple of days was separated from service. Sometime that summer, a group of us were sitting around when I suggested that perhaps we could play bridge. None of the rest knew the game so I volunteered to teach them. I took a pack of cards, shuffled them, and then found I couldn't remember a thing about how to play bridge, that is, I couldn't remember how many cards were dealt, if you drew for some cards — in short, absolutely nothing. I had to buy a book to recapture how to play bridge. I attributed this experience to essentially two factors: (1) a complete change of setting so that past associations with bridge had been completely cut off, and (2) the repression with which I dealt with my combat experiences.

During the period of military service, I had kept rather complete records of what I did. Later, in going through these diaries, I recalled the things that had happened to me, but in a very real sense I had intellectualized and isolated them from the associated affect. It was in a way as if I had never been in service at all. I recalled this as a way of explaining my sense of distance from things both of a personal and professional nature prior to my accident.

Dr. Gruenewald, of course, suspected that perhaps I had an ulterior motive in telling her of this episode. It became increasingly clear to me as we talked that I had never really experienced any real affective discharge toward this stroke. For the first six or seven weeks I had experienced no emotion at all, then later, until now, I had experienced momentary frustrations toward internal or external obstacles, but again, no ventilation regarding my disability. I had in a sense treated my whole accident as if I were sort of an experimental subject, an "object" for investigation rather than a person who had experienced a terrible trauma. It was a defense consistent with my identity as a professional person interested in research. Each person adapts to his organicity with his in-built psychological mechanisms.

The first session brought home to me the degree to which I had suppressed the situation. I was not a good hypnotic subject, as I might have suspected from studies having to do with the susceptibility of other operators. Nevertheless, I listened to Doris's induction procedures on hypnosis and tried to follow them, although it was very difficult not to intellectualize the situation. I succeeded in going into a very modest trance or at least a hypnoidal state. During this initial session, Doris asked me to go back to San Carlos and, through a projective hypnotic technique, inquired what I was doing. I thought of the house and pictured Bette and me working outside, planting flowers. I was immediately caught up in what it had meant for Bette and the children to move to Illinois. It was quite a concession for her to have to cut herself off from her friends and her home there. Very soon the tears were flowing. Bette and the children had given up so much to come here, primarily for the furthering of my professional career, which had now been cut short.

In the second session, Doris relinquished her attempts at hypnosis and placed the responsibility directly on me. Again, I have the feeling that I was partially successful in inducing self-hypnosis, although we spoke mostly of my professional activities with NIMH. I recalled that the night before I had had what might be called a posthypnotic dream. I was back working for NIMH and was busy looking through a list of research-approved grants, attempting to find out what happened to the grant of a colleague at the university. Then the scene was transformed and I was engaged in giving research consultation. I don't remember the details, but we were having an excellent time and I performed most adequately. This recalled in turn the first dream that I had had on February 27. In that dream I had accepted the fact that I was limited because of my stroke and had gone back to work at Fulton State Hospital (in Missouri). I was in charge of the psychology training program. Since I was unable to train people directly, because of my accident, I was looking through a file drawer of previous tapes that might be utilized for that purpose. We felt that the dream about NIMH was relatively positive in contrast to the earlier dream, which featured my acceptance of my disability.

Dr. Gruenewald had prepared a series of psychological tests based on my description of the areas in which I still suffered some deficit. On the day of my admission, I took a test battery in the waking condition and repeated it under hypnosis; but I do not think it was really successful. On Monday afternoon, prior to my departure from the hospital, I had a postexperimental battery. We tried hetero- and autohypnosis in relation to the test battery, but the effect, if any, soon wore off. In the EEG laboratory I attempted autohypnosis in lieu of drugs and surprisingly seemed to go to sleep without any medication. The lab technician at the time reported that I had been deeply asleep, but later in her written report of the examination stated that I was awake during the procedure, apparently because no medication was given to induce physiological sleep. The second EEG was essentially similar to the first. Six weeks later, a report from Doris on the psychological tests stated that there was no difference between the pre- and post-tests other than a slight positive finding on the post-test which could be attributable to a practice effect.

There is one other important event that bears mention in this brief period of hospitalization. I was interviewed by the ward psychiatrist, and in going over what had happened to me I recounted how the past and the future seemed to have lost all meaning for me. He dismissed this symptom as a variation of retrograde amnesia, although he admitted he had never heard a patient discuss the symptom quite as I had. In retrospect, I doubt very much that his conception could have been an explanation of what I had experienced. As I understand it, the victim either organically blots out or represses the specific circumstances surrounding the time of his accident and the immediate events leading up to it. My problem was exactly the opposite: I remembered in great detail the situation leading up to my accident and the trauma surrounding it. It was, in effect, an event that I remembered *too well* (even though I had no words to describe much of it at the time). The stroke acted as some sort of massive retroactive inhibition[2] which caused the gross dilution of all other experiences in my life.

Anyway, I came home from the hospital and for the next three weeks was deeply depressed. It was a most unusual depression for me since formerly I had tended to bounce back quickly from adversity. Bette was coming down with a cold and I did not tell her what had transpired except in very general terms. But when the depression lifted, the sense of distance from my past and future life was also gone. My life had become unified again! Somehow I connect my perception of the concept of *time* with this event. When I came to Illinois, I had an infinite amount of time to continue my professional career; after the accident, every minute was at a premium. It was as though in the instant of the accident I had been transformed from a very much alive, striving, professional person to a patient in a state of complete acceptance of death. Six months after the accident I still felt that if I could just interact in the next brief interpersonal exchange I would be thankful. I counted my objectives as measured by the hour, day, or, at most, a week.

---

[2] This is a psychological-experimental term which in learning theory means the intervention of a strident stimulus that causes preceding learned stimuli to be forgotten or repressed. Much later, I ran across the term "cultural shock" which seemed to me to capture at least part of the original sharp constriction. Cultural shock refers to a world that one can no longer make sense of nor understand. It designates the massive psychic reaction which takes place within the individual plunged into a culture vastly different from his own. It seemed that this to me is what a brain-injured person also goes through in attempting to make sense of his former (now foreign) life.

References

Greenberg, R., and Dewan, E. 1968. Aphasia and dreaming: a test of the P-hypothesis. *Psychophysiology,* 5, 203-04.

Jones, L. V., and Wepman, J. M. 1965. Aphasia research opens new insights into brain mechanisms. In *Research Projects Summaries* (No. 2), Bethesda: NIMH, pp. 69-77.

Kupper, H. I. 1945. Psychic concomitants in wartime injuries. *Psychosomatic Medicine,* 7, 15-21.

Moss, C. S. 1968. Experimental manipulation of dreams. In *Progress in Clinical Psychology* (ed. L. E. Abt and B. F. Reiss), New York: Grune and Stratton, 114-35.

2

Bette's Perception
of the Events

Upon my persistent urgings Bette finally sat down at the tape recorder in June of 1968 and dictated her memory of the accident seven months after it happened. I didn't listen to the tape for another six months, although I wouldn't maintain for a moment that these were independent observations. I think I sensed even then that my account of the initial stage of the accident was so clinical, detached and quite humorless — or at least it became manifest later on — that I wanted a much fuller account of the total impact of the stroke on my family. In a very real sense, my professionalism was against me in telling it in such a detached way — but this was my ultimate defense and quite obviously I could never have done it in any other way. Despite the effort to suppress it, the remembrances were still strong and frightening for my wife. This is her account of the episode and her very personal reactions to it. It coincides with my report but offers much more of the flavor of the effect of intense emotional upheaval upon the members of my family and what they were forced to go through.

BETTE: I often wonder if the move to Champaign had anything to do with the accident. I can remember our coming here in May [1967] and looking around at this flat farm land and saying, "Good heavens, we'd be out of our minds to leave California," even though we both had come from this area originally. And yet the opportunity to further

Scott's career was just too good to pass up, plus the fact that his traveling was getting a bit tiresome, and we needed a daddy home more
than he was. We got along all right and didn't complain, but it was
a difficult type of life. I always felt sorry for women who ended up
raising children by themselves and yet it almost bordered on this because on most weekdays the children and I were by ourselves much of
the time. It did look like a chance to have a different style of life,
snuggled into a little university town, and we didn't think we'd miss
the big city that much. But I suppose it was the opportunity of the
job itself which was most intriguing. There were compensations, we
told ourselves, but I think we can say that we somewhat reluctantly
agreed to leave the West Coast and come to Champaign.

There was the problem of selling the house [in San Carlos]. I worried
a great deal about that and it didn't seem that that went smoothly
at all. And then I suppose Scott's having to come on to Champaign
without us concerned me because of Joel's accident in which he
fell and broke his arm. The decision was made for us when the
orthopedist said that Joel could not travel for a month. So the kids
and I had to stay in San Carlos. We didn't get away until the third
of October, when Scott arrived. In the meantime we had packed the
house, our neighbors had packed the car, and the kids and I met Scott
at the airport and proceeded east. It was kind of exciting to be on
another new adventure, Joel was getting along O.K., and the little
ones were excited about the move. Actually we had a pleasant trip
east and everything went all right. We stopped in St. Louis for a
couple of days to see my dad, and then on to Champaign.

Scott had rented a "metal monstrosity," but the house certainly
looked like California and this helped us make the adjustment. So we
settled in and I remember thinking that I was so glad that Scott liked
to set up our various minor treasures which we had collected through
the years. He really has a knack for arranging things, which I suppose
is because of his art background. Anyway, I remember thinking that
I was so glad that he had taken over those built-in shelves in our
living room and put all those things on them because I'll bet I never
would have got that done with all that happened. So Scott pitched
right in and we managed to get the house livable.

We were there about a week when Scott had to go to Cincinnati for a meeting. I remember a couple of neighbors had asked us to come over for dessert, but he was gone and I didn't want to go without him. When Scott arrived in Cincinnati he called us, and just in that few short hours of the trip he had developed what seemed to be a terrific cold. He sounded very nasal, and his voice was quite husky the way it is when he gets a bad cold, but this seemed to have come on quite suddenly. Anyway, Scott didn't feel well, which was quite obvious. When he returned, he had what appeared to be a bad cold, and the coughing irritated us the most. I remember thinking that he should go see somebody about that cough, but I knew full well he wouldn't, having learned from past experience that he didn't really trust or believe in doctors for minor afflictions. The cough was so severe — he was up two or three hours a night for a week — but we still thought it was linked with just the cold. The following weekend we went to a dinner at Lloyd Humphreys' [chairman of the psychology department] and he didn't feel good then, although I don't remember that the coughing was too bad.

On that fateful night, October 30, he came home from the office and told me about his vision, and he suggested that it was only in the right eye, and for whatever reason I asked if he was certain that it was only in the one eye, and then he discovered it was actually in both eyes [as it turned out, the vision in the top half of *both* eyes refused to coincide with that in the bottom]. But how do you ever know about every illness that the human body is prone to develop unless you've experienced it or known someone who has? So there we were, ignorant of the whole thing. Even now, I don't know what we could have done, since finding out the inadequacies of the local physicians. I really think that in this instance ignorance was bliss. We might have suspected, as now I think we should have, that something was going wrong inside his brain. But if we had, who knows whom we would have got hold of, and anybody we might have called could have messed up the whole thing, so I guess to make me feel better I think it was well that we didn't suspect a stroke.

Anyway, Scott's headache that evening should have told us something, but we just didn't realize what in the world was going on. We think now that the cough had to do with the closing of the artery, but then we just didn't know, I suppose because Scott had always been so healthy, and outside of gaining weight in the winter which he lost in the summer he was in good physical health. When I think back on it, the one time that I did persuade Scott to go see "Uncle George" (we called him that because he had a long-sounding Greek name), he recommended that Scott go for further tests to the hospital. But Scott never did go because the trouble subsided and he was too busy traveling.

I don't like to have to go back and remember all this. People kept asking me, how did I know what to do? The answer was I didn't know what to do and I don't know that what I did was right. You don't stop and think at times like this. I saw him fall, and I still thought he was teasing because once in a while when we would kid each other Scott would stagger around. So I wanted to think that was what he was doing this time, but obviously he wasn't. He didn't stop coughing until he fell down, and then the coughing abruptly stopped. He was still reaching for that blamed TV just to watch the dumb Packers! He fell down on his knees and elbows, and I could see he was trying to get up and couldn't. He looked at me with a cockeyed smile where one side of his face didn't move; then of course I knew that something was terribly wrong. I was frightened and I was going to run to do something. I got the operator and asked her to send an ambulance. I didn't know what else to do, I didn't know any neighbors, and it was almost 11:30 at night. Scott was so hot, beads of perspiration stood out on his head. He kept trying to get up and kept looking at me, almost pleading with me to do something, but I didn't know what to do. He apparently could not talk. I simply tried to keep him quiet, which he was.

It wasn't long before the ambulance arrived. It was raining outside. It was a very nice man who came in and asked me where they should take him. I had no answer to this, but I remembered seeing a large medical center and that's where I thought we should go. The men were very, very nice, and asked if I wanted to go with them. I couldn't because our three children were asleep, but I promised to come over as soon as I could get someone to stay with the children. At this point I called Don Peterson. I told him something had happened to Scott, that I didn't know what, but that I'd had him taken to the hospital. I was in my pajamas at the time so I went in and got dressed and it didn't take Don fifteen minutes to get to the house. I don't remember what we said to each other; I was close to hysterics because I was so frightened and I didn't know what had happened, except I felt the world had suddenly caved in on us. First he said he would take me to the hospital, but I insisted I could drive myself, so he said he would stay with the children. The ambulance driver had called me in the meantime to say that they had my husband in the emergency room and did I know where it was. I said I would find it.

When I arrived, Scott was still in the emergency room. No one was in there with him, no doctor or anyone, he was simply lying on this cart. I don't know how long we waited but it was a heck of a long time for the doctor to arrive. It seems to me he didn't get there until about 1:30 A.M. He was an internist who happened to be on call. By this time the paralysis had left Scott's arm and leg. The doctor did the usual tapping and listening, and then he said, "Tell me what happened." I thought Scott couldn't talk, so I went through the account of what I thought had happened. And then he turned and said to Scott, "Now you tell me." And Scott spoke up and told him in effect what I had told him. I remember being surprised that he could talk and so fluently. Occasionally he'd block, but for the most part he gave the same ac-counting that I did. The doctor said that he didn't know what had happened, but he suggested that Scott stay the night and maybe they'd run a couple of tests on him the next day.

At that juncture Scott was wheeled up to pediatrics since they didn't have any other empty beds. They put him in a little room off in the corner and I stayed with him until about 3 A.M. The only thing I noticed while I was still there was that while Scott could talk to me, he was very cold, he had the chills, and I remember asking for blankets and heaping them on his bed. But he was still quite cold and I don't remember now how long that lasted. We agreed that possibly he should try to sleep and he actually dozed a little bit. I wasn't worried about his speech at all since we had engaged in considerable conversation. I then called Don at home and told him that I just about had him settled down, and I suppose I got back about 3:30 A.M. It's funny, too, I've often thought, that surely somewhere in the psychological studies one must have come across symptoms of a stroke, and yet trying to explain to Don how Scott appeared and what had happened, he didn't evidence any knowledge as to what had happened either.

In the morning, knowing they were going to run these tests, I called the hospital about 9 A.M. after sending the children off to school. I didn't tell Scott's mother he was in the hospital, since I didn't want to alarm her unnecessarily. The girl who answered the phone said that Dr. Moss was in having some tests run and she would have him call me when he came back. So I went on about what I was doing. I eventually called again and she said yes, he was in his room and she would put him on. She apparently gave Scott the phone and he uttered a sound but that's all that it was; I could not make head or tail out of what he was trying to say to me. I remember feeling that I had just fallen down to China. My heart just dropped! And there he was just babbling something over the phone to me, but nothing that I could understand. At this juncture I knew that something was very wrong and I simply said to him, "Well, let's hang up the phone and I'll be there in a few minutes." I got over there as quickly as I could, and when I saw him he could say absolutely nothing to me. He just looked at me. Apparently he understood me but he couldn't say anything back. And as so often happens there were no doctors around to tell me anything. The nurses were in and out but I don't think they understood what was going on with Scott.

I remember sitting by his bed (by this time he had been moved into a double room), and I would talk to him and he'd just look at me. I'd try to get him to even answer questions where he could shake his head yes or no. He seemed to understand what I said. I guess I was simply not letting myself think that something was really that wrong with him. I just would not accept that. And so he and I played little games where I would try to get him to say different things. I'd repeat the alphabet, slowly, A — and he'd say "A"; and I'd say B — and he'd say "Beh"; and then I'd get on to D, and he'd say "A" again. That was all that I could get him to do, repeat A, B, C. He'd smile when he did this though, and whether he couldn't say the D or he simply didn't care — he was like a child who wanted to play games. So that's what we did while I was there with Scott — play games.

I remember mistakenly thinking, well, maybe he could write

something to me. I'd say to him when I left, "Do you want me to bring you something? Can I bring you something to eat?" — because he wasn't eating anything. And he'd nod his head "yes." Then I'd say, "Well, what is it you want?" And then he'd babble something which I couldn't understand. And finally I decided that maybe Scott could write to me. So I gave him a pencil and a paper and asked him to write it down. I wish now that I had saved some of the things that he wrote to me, but I didn't have the foresight to save them. Of course what he wrote wasn't even letters, it was just little discrete markings. Eventually I began playing a game like Twenty Questions with him, in response to what he wanted. We always got around to a milkshake every time. So I'd stop downstairs on my way up and order a chocolate milkshake for him. He'd act as though he wanted it and maybe he'd take one or two swallows and then leave the rest.

I knew they had called in a neurologist but I never laid eyes on the man all the time Scott was in the hospital. The internist was rather vague, too. I knew they had run a series of tests on him, but after waiting until the second day I called the neurologist's office and received a runaround from the receptionist. I gave her half an hour and then called her back. I demanded to know what these tests were, that I was his wife and had a right to know what they'd found out. She replied that the neurologist had placed the results in a file and turned it over to the internist. At this point I called him and he wasn't there, so I left word for him to call me as soon as possible. At the end of that day, at 10 o'clock, he finally called and reported that they thought Scott had a primary brain tumor which meant it was operable or he had cancer that had begun in his lungs and had spread to his brain, and if this was so there was nothing they could do about it. They left me with those two choices for another day! It was unbearable; I almost went out of my mind — yet trying not to let Scott know that *I* knew there could be anything this wrong.

But Scott was in such a happy mood — he really didn't care one way or the other — he was in no pain. He dozed most of the time, or when I was there we'd play our little game or I'd talk to him and he'd listen and smile and act as though he understood. I'd say things like "Who am I? Do you know me?" And he'd nod his head "yes." And then I'd say, "Am I your sister?" No, I wasn't his sister. He acted as though he knew who I was. And then I'd say, "Do you have any children?" He'd indicate that he did. Then I'd say, "How many children do you have?" Sometimes he'd indicate four and sometimes five (we actually have three). And I never knew exactly but I still think that he didn't lose his sense of humor, because we've always played that way with each other. I think he was still displaying a sense of humor, which is just incredible. I knew perfectly well he really knew how many children he had — that he was simply playing with me.

Finally the internist called again on the third night and said there was no cancer of the lungs and they had decided that it was a primary brain tumor. His remark to me was that he would strongly suggest that I take him to Chicago because there was nobody here that he would let touch a member of his family. Well, that decided it for me — we would take him to Chicago. They subsequently made a referral to Presbyterian–St. Luke's and to Dr. Oldberg and his staff. We went two days later. I had the children to consider too, and Jean Peterson was marvelous, she did her best to find someone to come in and take care of them. I also had to tell the children about daddy and to try to explain to a five-, seven- and ten-year-old where we were going. When we came back from Chicago, I discovered how the older boy's school work had suffered. Joel is a quiet boy. He has feelings but they often aren't demonstrable, he hides them well, and really, in all the worry and concern about Scott, I thought the children were all right. As I found out later, his school work fell considerably. He was much more aware of the danger and the trouble we were in than I had realized.

The night that I found out what they thought at the hospital about a tumor was the first time I called my father in St. Louis and told him Scott was in the hospital. I didn't tell him too much about it except for the diagnosis and the fact that I was taking him to Chicago. He listened to me, of course, and asked what he could do. I said, "Nothing that I know of." He said not to worry about money because he would help out on that, and I knew he would if we needed it. But then the next morning he called back and of course he had had all evening to think about this, and he said he wanted to go to Chicago with me. "I can't bear to think of you going through this and being all alone." And when he said "all alone" my fears mounted and that was the beginning of the shaking up, because, going back a bit, of all the heartaches he has had in his life and some in mine — we had seen my little nephew operated on for what supposedly was a brain tumor, and as a result he was physically and intellectually maimed — so a brain operation was not exactly new to either of us and we knew what would lie ahead if the surgery was to take place. So Dad and I must have had this in the back of our minds. I remember crying very hard after I hung up the phone; he was feeling the same way I was — feeling for me.

I sat down with the children the night before we left and attempted to tell them that daddy was very ill, because at this point I thought he was going to have surgery. But this threatened my control — I didn't want to break down in front of the children. Up until now I had managed to hold myself together pretty well, probably because I still refused to believe that anything was going to happen to him. I saw him and I knew he was sick and that something was drastically wrong, but I would not accept the fact that he wouldn't be all right again. This is what held me together.

I also finally had to tell Scott's mother what was happening. I told her first that Scott had had this bad cough and I'd taken him to the hospital, still trying to spare her the hurt and the anxiety of knowing all this. When eventually I had to tell her, I hoped that she would stay with the children, but she said no, she wasn't up to staying with the children and she wanted to go to Chicago, too. So a young couple, he was an assistant professor here and they had no children, volunteered at the last minute to come in and live in the house, so that part of the problem was resolved. I called them every night after getting back from the hospital. Don Peterson made arrangements for us to stay at student housing in Chicago, and we took taxis back and forth.

The morning we left to go it was snowing. We had a very nice ambulance driver again and Scott's mother sat up in front with him while I sat in back by Scott. He was extremely quiet, of course, during the whole trip. I kept asking him if he was all right. He just sort of dozed — he didn't notice anything going on about him. We went right into Presbyterian–St. Luke's hospital and they got him settled in his room. Then the team came in, led by Dr. Matz, a resident

neurosurgeon. I never did see Dr. Oldberg. Scott said later that he
saw him once, when he was leading a group of interns; they looked
him over for maybe five minutes. I remember when Matz came in to
see him for the first time, I was sort of surprised that Scott mobilized
himself to answer Matz's questions with "yes" and "no." At least he
could understand him, but that was apparently the limit of his
vocabulary at this time.

When we arrived at Presbyterian–St. Luke's it was on Friday,
the beginning of the weekend. I knew they didn't run tests in hospitals
on Saturday or Sunday, but I felt that time was of the essence. Dr.
Matz did say that no one would be around on the weekend, and I
asked if time didn't have something to do with Scott's condition, and
why in the world would they let him lie there for two days before they
did anything. So he said he would have some tests run Saturday.
But I guess if I hadn't said anything, Scott would have just waited
until Monday. The doctor did give him a preliminary examination,
and there is the possibility he knew there was no urgency, but his
thoughts weren't shared with me if such was the case.

They ran their own independent studies, which included an angiogram. They also called in a vascular team. At this point they discovered
that the left artery was blocked and that surgery was not possible.
They in effect could do nothing for him. They announced that time
was the biggest element in his eventual recovery, whatever that might
be. There was no medication given and they had no suggestions to
make whatsoever. Of course Scott lost considerable weight. I also lost
weight because of anxiety. Mother and I would go through the
motions of trying to eat a meal or two but it didn't work very well.

As if we didn't have enough to think about, I also became ill with
a hormone upset and had to seek out a gynecologist to get myself
straightened out. It just added to the discomfort all the way around.
Mostly our days were just spent going over to the hospital as soon
as we were allowed in and sitting with him all day. I used to attempt
to feed him when his lunch or dinner came but there wasn't much
that he wanted to eat. I'd bring him a milkshake, and sometimes
he'd drink a bit of that but not much. Drink was all that he did want,
he wouldn't eat a meal at all. He was just content to lie in bed.
We'd get the newspapers and I'd try to tell him what was going on.

We also had a TV in the room and I turned on a football game or two; he looked at it some but I doubt that he was really interested.

I am reminded of something that happened in the hospital — he used to do things like this every now and then, even during the height of his illness. It is one of the things that really kept me going. In the hospital he wasn't saying anything but simply listening to me and watching me, and I got up from the chair by his bed to leave the room, and he patted me on the fanny. I turned around quickly and looked at him and there was that familiar twinkle in his eye, and I knew that I still had the same Scott I started with. I don't care what his outward appearance was, he was still basically the same person. This is another reason why I refused to believe that anything really, really could be wrong with him.

Our friends the Noltes dropped in from Decatur; we met them one night in the elevator when we were coming down to get something to eat. I was very glad to see them. Mary is a dear person; she had her nurse's uniform with her and was all set to stay and nurse Scott if we needed her. I'll never forget that Mary did this. When John and Mary came to the hospital, I sent them up to Scott's room, but I said that they shouldn't expect Scott to say anything although I was sure he would like to see them and would enjoy their talking to him. But after they did go on, I was quite nervous because I thought he wouldn't want me to have sent anyone up when he couldn't talk to them and I wasn't there. I felt a strong urge to run back to the room to protect him from being in that situation, feeling that he might be quite upset with me for having done this. But we went on and had a quick bite to eat anyway, and when we got back to the room he was just lying there smiling at them. They were sort of making small talk, and apparently it wasn't bothering him a bit to have them there. He didn't mind that he couldn't talk to them. I felt a great sense of relief.

There were many, many phone calls that came in on the phone by the bed. People called from all over to find out about him. The word had spread very quickly. I had called our friends the Scanderups in San Carlos to tell Dorothy and Dean about the accident and I asked them to call the Federal Building in San Francisco to inquire about whether Scott was still covered by federal group insurance.

This immediately prompted a phone call from John Bell, the director of the mental health operation in the region, so the word got out, not only through neighbors in San Carlos but through NIMH in Washington. So calls were coming in constantly from people who knew Scott from all over. He had been doing so well in his field, and then to have this crashing blow — everybody felt for him and their concern was genuine; I really did appreciate it. When I would sit by his bed and repeat the name of the person, he would seem to know who it was and I would know he understood what I was saying to him.

They didn't tell me what was actually wrong with him until the evening before we went home. When they finally did tell me, they still said they were going to keep him a couple of days, and I said, "No, you're not! I want to get out of here in the morning, so sign us out; Scott is going to go home. If there is nothing you can do for him here, I can do a lot more at home. I can feed him and do exactly the same things and more than you're doing here." Dr. Matz was very nice and said he would try, and I said, "You do more than try, you get us out of here!" So he did. That evening I called Don Peterson and asked if he could get someone to drive our car up, because I didn't want to come back in the ambulance. Don did get a graduate student and his wife to drive up and get us. So we brought him home. The couple who had stayed with our children wouldn't take anything — she told me I would spoil everything they had done if I persisted in wanting to pay her. They had taken good care of the children and we were really most grateful for this.

We tried to reestablish some sort of a normal life — as normal as it could be. The children were glad to see daddy back, of course, and I remember all of them coming up and hugging him and trying to ask him things. Of course he didn't answer. I had to say to them that they should talk to daddy, and that though he might not want to talk, he would listen and understand what they were saying. I tried to tell them not to expect him to talk a lot to them, without trying to explain why he couldn't talk. They really accepted it very well, and they'd play little games with him, too. They were very good about it. As he got to where he could say a few words after some weeks, he would likely as not say things wrong, and they'd just laugh. We'd all laugh, including Scott. It wasn't anything that they minded at all — they just thought it was kind of funny and joked about it.

I tried to get some weight back on him — he was quite thin — and eventually he began to eat a little bit. He'd try to read the newspaper but he couldn't. I don't remember how long it was before he really talked much to me. I guess I became aware that he wasn't interested in anything. I ran the house and did all the things that had to be done, and he was like a star boarder. He ate and slept at our house but without much interaction. He was pleasant. Actually I thought, in the beginning, that he couldn't be taking this as well as he appeared to be. He understood what was wrong, and I would think, knowing him, that he should be very angry and upset over this turn of events, but he wasn't. He just accepted it and I suppose that this was all part of it. He really didn't care that much about anything. He didn't think about it, as I know now, so how could he be worried about it. In the beginning I thought he would be in a miserable mood all of the time and very irritated, but of course he wasn't. He was like a very pleasant guy who was just there. He'd eat as well as he could whatever I'd fix him and he'd sit and watch TV or just sit.

But it wasn't long before he decided that he was going to get busy. For example, he was going to try to read his professional journals, which was extremely difficult for him. He would pick up a journal and try to read something, but it didn't last long — he just couldn't keep the thoughts together. It seemed to go better if I would read to him. I spent all of my time with him, except getting meals, doing washing and ironing, and taking care of the children. But the rest of the time we spent together, talking, and trying to regain whatever we could that seemed to have been lost. He had no memory for past events. He knew vaguely that we had been in California, but he didn't remember people, even people that we really knew well. Perhaps he could picture them in his mind when I introduced the names, but he sure couldn't remember anybody's name, not a single person, even people that lived next door or people that he worked with. I would try to recall incidents that we had experienced or laughed about but he often didn't appear to recall them. His whole past seemed to have been wiped out. He was, in some ways, a cabbage, but not really.

I remember the first time that Lloyd Humphreys came over, someone whom he was very self-conscious about in his situation, which is one thing that I always felt was wrong in his attitude, and yet I couldn't expect him to act in any other way. He's always been a perfectionist so he was no different about this than anything else. He wasn't ashamed of what had happened but he seemed to feel that he had no right to act the way he was. He should try to act normally. I always felt that this was wrong. If you've had an accident it's not any fault of yours, and if you can't respond to something because of this, this is not any fault of yours. And why in the world did he have to put up some kind of a front and try to pretend that he was better than he was — but this is the difference in the way we look at things. If something like this had happened to me and my friends or associates came around, I could only act a certain way and I wouldn't try to act any differently. But he felt so bad for having had this happen to him — he just wouldn't accept the fact that something had happened in the brain that simply would not allow him to talk any better at the time.

But returning to Lloyd, I remember the three of us sat in the living room and we had a drink. Lloyd chatted away and Scott did his best to try to converse with him, but felt very ill at ease the whole time that Lloyd was there. I really didn't think that Lloyd expected him to do anything outstanding — after all, unless you've had it happen to you, you don't understand it (and we eventually found out Lloyd's mother had had a stroke and suffered from mild aphasia). No one expected Scott to do an outstanding job in anything but he seemed to feel that they expected him to. You can only do what you can and no one had any right to expect otherwise.

For the most part my feelings were, even at this time, that he would come out of this, that we'd work at it as we could, and actually at the beginning there was rapid improvement, and this brings us around to the positive side of perfectionism. I think if he had just sat and not tried to do anything his improvement would not have been as rapid — he pushed himself hard to do things. I think it is very good that he did it this way, that he wanted to do it this way. He was committed to writing a couple of articles and there was a deadline coming up on one of them. I felt that I had done a pretty good job of holding us together until this time and because he hadn't been angry about anything it had been rather pleasant, all things considered. But when we began to work on this article for the first time he became extremely angry with himself, and then began to shout at me. This is the first and possibly the only time when I felt sorry for myself. Having feelings of my own, I felt he didn't need to yell at me, but it only lasted a little while, and then I realized that it was a selfish thing for me to feel this way. After all, he couldn't help how he was acting under the pressure to begin speaking again. So I got over it quickly, and we went on working on the article. It was very difficult for me to try to understand what he was attempting to say to me. I guess I had read enough of what he had written and typed enough of his manuscripts so that I was a little familiar with his terminology. I could pick out what he would write in contrast to something written by another, that is, his style of writing, so I guess all of this helped me to try to put down what he was saying. But it was extremely difficult; as much as I wanted to help do it, it got to the point where I dreaded these sessions. It seemed to take so much out of him and it made me irritable too.

Even before the accident happened he would get angry at himself and would occasionally take it out on me, and this was always upsetting to me. I don't like to see people angry, I don't like to be around people who are angry, we don't like to be around couples who are constantly bickering. So when somebody gets angry at me it is very upsetting to me, although in this instance I should have realized why he was angry. He wasn't angry at me — he was angry at himself. Anyway, we stuck to the manuscript, mailed it off, and they did accept the paper, which was just marvelous for us. From then on we began writing a little bit more. He worked on more and more, and I really think that being the type of person that he was, he was fortunate in this kind of an accident, because I don't know whether somebody else would have begun to work as soon as he did and would have kept at it as hard as he did. I feel that this was Scott doing this, not just a patient — it was his own personality that drove him so hard to get himself well. A lot of people would have given up or at the very least it would have taken them some time before they had the motivation to try to work and to force themselves to talk and read and understand.

Here is a note that Julie wrote about that time describing her recollection of the accident and the impression it had upon her:

My father had an accident not long ago and this is what I remember. It all happened at night when I was asleep so in the morning I went downstairs and Mom was crying. I asked her what was the matter? She said, "Daddy is sick and in the hospital." Well, I told her everything was going to be all right and said, "Please stop crying."

And then she went away to the hospital and the Clowers [Clores] stayed with us at our house. The next thing I remember is Mom came home with Dad. They came home and when Daddy stepped in the door he looked at us kids, he looked in sort of half surprise and half confused. Well, we hugged him and he said, "Hullow."

Now he stalls to think of words and his temper is much shorter. Sometimes he wants to call me and he says, "Kevin, ah Joel, ah Julie." But no matter how acward he ever gets, we still love him just the same.

When Scott was here taking his graduate work, he happened to take a course under Joseph Wepman, who is one of the few experts in the country on aphasia. So he decided he wanted to go and talk to Joe. I set up an appointment with him. One cold morning Scott and I got on the train and had a nice trip into Chicago. It was enjoyable because we were hopeful that if anyone could help Scott it was Dr. Wepman. He could give Scott recommendations about what to do to improve. We had lunch first at the International House on the Chicago campus, where Scott lived during his internship. He showed me around a bit and we really had a nice time. Then we spent the afternoon with Dr. Wepman's assistants and they did some tests on him. I didn't talk to anybody then. We went home with the information that they would rerun the tests three weeks later. Anyway, Scott enjoyed seeing Joe and we both felt that maybe they would help him.

Then we went back again and at this point they talked with me, too. They retested Scott and in the three weeks' time they felt they saw a great deal of improvement, and this is the way we felt, too, because the improvement was very rapid at this time. But what it all boiled down to was Dr. Wepman telling him that there really wasn't anything that he could do to speed up the recovery, and that given a few more months or so he would probably be fully recovered and he would be very interested in seeing Scott at that time. So this buoyed our spirits considerably. I remember the train ride back on the Panama Limited and our sitting in the club car. We had a drink and then went back to the diner and had a nice dinner. We were just floating on clouds because we took to heart what Dr. Wepman had said to us and we really felt that in another couple of months Scott would be entirely recovered. Unfortunately, the prediction didn't turn out to be correct.

Scott continues to improve day by day but gradually the improvement has begun to slow down. It is no longer quite so spectacular, although I still see improvement in the various areas. For instance, at first he couldn't type at all, but he has stuck to it and little by little he types a little faster, with plenty of errors, but he remembers where to put his fingers. Probably the thing that has stayed the worst has been his handwriting, but before the accident his handwriting wasn't anything to brag about. I think that even that has improved a bit. He still finds that when he talks to people he cannot follow long, involved conversations. For his part, Scott can talk for a few minutes and everything's fine, but he simply needs time to put his words in order. If it gets to be an extended conversation, he is likely to lose the area of thought. And he can't take notes because he can't write that well.

No one had advised Scott to take any speech therapy; in fact, Dr. Wepman was against it, but Scott has gone to the speech department. It certainly can't hurt him any and it gives him a chance to talk to people other than me, because he is extremely self-conscious about talking to anyone else. He feels that he might make a mistake and then he'd block, and he doesn't want to do this. He just can't stand the fact that he doesn't talk exactly the way he used to. I'm constantly saying, "But people don't expect you to talk like you used to," and he'll end up getting angry with me. The point is that he wants to talk the way he remembers and he isn't going to have it any other way. If he can't talk that way, then he isn't going to talk! So there!

3

Recovery at Twelve Months

In November of 1968 I summarized the daily log on my progress to date in the following way.

It has been a year since my accident. My family and I agree that I still continue to progress, although the improvement has gradually slackened. What residuals of my stroke am I aware of?

I used to be more or less continually happy. In the morning, I usually awoke humming a little tune and generally the adverse events of the day did not bother me for long. That optimistic edge was taken away by my stroke, or, more precisely, rightly or not I attributed this partially to my medication. Presbyterian–St. Luke's prescribed nothing for me when I left the hospital; however, a neurologist whom I saw for a single visit two months later prescribed a recently developed anticoagulant, which I began taking twice a day. I took the pills for over eight months, never realizing that I should see any physician about possible side effects. One consequence was that during this entire period I was relatively depressed. On the other hand, let me be fair and admit that the confounding factor was that this was the period of my greatest readjustment. When I gave up the anticoagulant my mood seemed to brighten somewhat, so I can render this only as a highly subjective judgment.[1]

---

[1] Bette writes: "We were advised to get in touch with a local neurologist and we went down to see him one day. He had made the original diagnosis, and he of course didn't say anything about that, but he did apologize to us for not

I still find it difficult to write (agraphia) — after a few words
or a sentence or two, my handwriting deteriorates rapidly. Similarly,
my typing became abominable after the accident, but now is slowly
improving, more than my handwriting. The trouble is that my writing
is very labored and my thoughts soon outstrip it. As I fall further
behind, I try to speed up the handwriting and thus it becomes completely illegible. The typewriter does a better job, although I notice
that I have difficulty sustaining adequate pressure with right-hand keys.
I end up with the left-hand letters being firmly imprinted, and the
right-hand letters serving as sort of "shadows" to them. The most
familiar analogy that I can give is that it is vaguely similar to the
experience of writer's cramp. My difficulty in writing and typing is
naturally a holdover from the original paralysis. In contrast, my
ability to play ping-pong has not suffered the same disability — which
testifies to the exquisite visual-motor coordination in writing.

Where I suffer in writing the most is in making mnemonic notes to
myself in formal group settings. For years I had the habit of making
cryptic little notes to speak from; now I can't do this, which, in
combination with my spotty memory, makes speaking a hazardous
affair at best. (I have toyed around with the idea of taking some kind
of simplified shorthand.) Also I still have some difficulty in reading

---

having run these tests himself ('We have all of the equipment here but not
anybody to run them'). I can't be convinced that even had the tests been run that
he would have known how to read them. He prescribed an anticoagulant for
Scott and while on it Scott seemed to be depressed. His days had been 'ups' and
'downs'; some days were good, but on other days he would start out feeling good
but almost as quickly as you could snap your fingers he'd go into a depression.
But when he was on the anticoagulant he seemed depressed most of the time,
although we didn't realize what was causing it.

"Our social life was nil, or almost so, but a couple of times we would go
to some gathering of the psychology faculty. Scott would go if there was a large
group of people, which meant he wouldn't be required to talk much. You can
pretty much just listen when you're around a big group of people, especially if
the group has had a bit to drink, because everyone wants to talk. That's when
we ran into one of the psychology wives who had had some heart problems
causing her to go into the hospital. Her physician advised her to take this same
anticoagulant, but she refused because of all the side effects. When she told us
this, Scott took it upon himself to discontinue taking the anticoagulant; immediately he began to feel better and the depression was lifted. This is just another
example of the frustration we felt from lack of reliable medical knowledge."

(alexia). I read the newspaper or magazines such as *Time* or *Life* now without any appreciable difficulty, at least the shorter articles, but textbooks or journal articles are much more time-consuming than formerly. High-level conceptions take more time and I rather quickly tire of that level of reading or communication.

Most mention here has been of my problems in expressive speaking or writing, and I presume that this part of my communication system suffered the most; however, I also suffer difficulties in receptive intake or comprehension of what is said or written. This was most apparent immediately following the stroke, especially where the messages were multiple and/or came at too fast a rate. When I returned to the clinic, for example, I attended all of the weekly staff meetings religiously, and I tried hard to listen carefully and make sense out of what was being said, but so many people's verbalizations invariably stupefied me. Trying to follow each person's contribution, to integrate the various topics, and also attempting to formalize what I might say in response was just too taxing, and after a while I inevitably lapsed back into a semiconscious reverie.

Fortunately, this situation has greatly improved; at least now I can follow most of what is said, only I still cannot make any sort of rejoinder, because by the time that I have put my thoughts into words, the conversation has drifted well beyond that point. This is somehow related to the fact that I feel most confident on the phone, or in individual conversations, where I have only one person to relate to. It is reminiscent of the feelings that I still have when I go to any of the shopping centers. I become rapidly inundated by the plethora of incoming stimuli — it is almost more than I can assimilate — I actually get to feeling dizzy after a few minutes. There is nothing wrong with my vision, I might add. I recently had a complete eye examination, including an eye field scan, and nothing unusual could be detected.

One other thing while I think of it — if I don't stop to think before I give directions, I am quite likely to confuse myself or other people by getting left mixed up with right or vice versa. In close-order drill I would really be a Gomer Pile. This indicates some damage to the parietal lobe, which again may or may not be related to a common error in writing. More often than not I now interchange letters or occasionally words. Similarly, if I miss a word in typing and later discover it, there is a definite tendency in replacing the missing word to put it slightly earlier than it should occur. All such errors occur automatically. If I stop and think I can usually catch such mistakes even before they happen, but this makes it very difficult to function spontaneously.

Basically, the main problem is that I block on words and I am still "shocked" into silence by my inability to find appropriate words. I often fall silent rather than say what I know will be an inappropriate word. I still stumble on even the most pedestrian words. In fantasy I sometimes pretend that my accident never happened or that if it did, I am fully recovered, but I am brought back to reality by the very next relationship. To put it another way, my "inner speech" seems to have made a partial recovery, and when I block on a word this reflects that I am still blocked internally, that is, the instant I know a word, then I can say it. This points up another thing, that thinking is not speech or vice versa. They are distantly related cousins but for the most part my perception is that I am more capable of thinking things through than in explaining them in words. They are decidedly not the same thing.

My ability to capture appropriate words seems affected by either anxiety or fatigue. In connection with the former, I do find inter-personal relationships extremely tiring, particularly with professional contacts. With my colleagues, I am frequently at a loss to specify a necessary conception, while at the same time I feel that I must measure each word precisely to make certain that it communicates the exact meaning that I intend it to have. The upshot is that the process of searching for words defeats me, and I then have the definite tendency to withdraw from professional and even social contacts.[2]

---

[2] Bette again writes: "We had done a lot of entertaining when we were in California and enjoyed it, and knowing that university people make their own entertainment more or less, we looked forward to this, too. All of this was drastically curtailed with the accident. We went over to Don and Jean's one night and they had the Weirs over, too. Cecelia wanted us to come over for dinner, so with some reluctance Scott agreed to go. It turned out to be one other couple and us, and Scott was extremely quiet while there and this bothered him. I'm sure he felt ill at ease the whole time and I felt bad because of him. Then as soon as we had eaten dinner we sat down in the living room to talk. It couldn't have been more than five minutes later when Scott indicated to me

With my own children, where I am relatively relaxed, the opposite is true. I am liable to slur my speech or even to engage in word-finding difficulty or occasional neologisms (i.e. I frequently call one of them by the other's name or ask them if they want to go to the Antifreeze rather than the Dairy Queen, or request them to get into their BVD's when I mean swimming suits, or, when hurried, may actually use a term which is a nonword — a nonsense syllable). My children seem to take it in stride, laughing in good nature at a particularly peculiar mal-use of words.

Actually, my work day spans more or less the same length of time as formerly — about sixteen to seventeen hours. I do not tire easily doing physical chores, and I am relieved to know that at least I still have much of the physical stamina that I had formerly. I swim, wrestle with the children, bowl, and play ping-pong — and I am apparently in excellent physical health. I took a policy with an insurance company about three months ago, and the examining physician could detect no physical or psychological deficiencies at all (I gauged my conversation with the doctor very carefully, of course). The company did increase my rate by 25 percent for the next eight years, so I infer that actually I am not on my actuarial deathbed yet. My overriding objective is to make my family's life financially secure, not in the event of death but in the event of another totally disabling "accident."

I felt it was extremely important to reestablish and strengthen the emotional ties with my family. In the summer of 1968 we purchased a home in a newly developed subdivision and in many ways it has been highly therapeutic for me to have to attend to so many household duties. Joel, our ten-year-old son, has made Little League again this summer, and my wife and I attended each of his games. All three

that he wanted to go home. I felt bad for having eaten and then immediately left. I felt they would understand but from then on we didn't go to any more gatherings like that, because I realized what a horrible strain it was on Scott. People at the university knew what had happened to him and we didn't get invitations after a while, and if we did get invited to a party, we usually turned it down. After being used to an active social life it is hard to get adjusted to being alone, but any attempt to socialize was simply not worth it. For a while I had the urge to have someone in for dinner or the evening, but the strain on Scott simply made it not worth doing. I think we've become partly acclimated and I really don't miss it much any more."

of the children were enrolled in summer school. Their schedules varied and this necessitated a more or less continuous taxi service. My wife's observation is that I now enjoy the children as much or more than I ever did.

Through the past ten years (long before my stroke), I held to the fantasy that someday, happily, I might develop some sort of an innocuous illness, like a mild case of t.b., that would force me to bed for a year or so, and give me the time to catch up on all of the professional journals and books which attracted my attention, but for which I simply had no time. Instead, I ended up with a health complication that prohibits me from indulging in most intellectual pursuits.

Consciously, I vaguely feared a heart attack as I approached a very active middle age, but at the same time I suspect that I actually feared damage to my intelligence. I had no trouble sleeping, but once in a great while I had what could be considered a nightmare, and three or four of these had a common theme. In 1952, for example, I had had a dream in which I was a patient in a psychiatric hospital. I was sitting in the canteen with some of my friends, but due to the fact that I had received a series of convulsive shocks, I was completely unable to converse with them. I awoke from the dream feeling panicky but was immensely relieved to find that it was only fantasy. In my wildest imagination I have wondered, these days, could there be a homunculus who directed that the clot would end up in my head rather than my heart, and thus deprive me of the time that I would devote to reading and thinking?

Actually it has rather astonished me that I have withstood the acute and later the nonflagging stress of severe brain damage as well as I did, without resorting to various neurotic defenses or to depression or even worse. Perhaps it is only because I was sensitized to numerous cases of acute and chronic brain syndromes in persons who had developed psychiatric symptoms that I was predisposed to expect that I too would develop a more morbid disorder. For example, I found my memory drawn back to a patient that I had seen almost fifteen years earlier, whom I must have unconsciously partially identified with. The patient was middle aged at the time, married, and formerly employed as a professor of mechanical engineering, who had undergone numerous deleterious personality changes since removal of a tumor from the right frontal lobe five years before. Whereas formerly he had been reported as exceedingly capable, industrious, and sociable, he had become irascible, garrulous, and captious — behavior which confounded every one of his interpersonal relationships, and finally resulted in his confinement at a hospital.

I remember attempting to work with the patient in psychotherapy for some months, but he was without insight into the seriousness of his condition, and I couldn't breach his absolute denial. The patient lacked entirely any sensitivity in his interpersonal relationships, his tolerance for frustration was extremely low, and when exceeded (as it was several times a session) he would react in an agitated and rigid manner, although he was not physically assaultive. He made frequent defensive protests of his own personal superiority and was hypercritical and tactless in dealing with others; for example, he was very verbal about the ignorance and deceit of the members of the staff who kept him hospitalized, and he wrote dozens of letters to local, state, and even national officials excoriating them over his unjust imprisonment. The point is that I was worried about such cases on the basis of possible self-reactions to my own disorder, but apparently this was a gross misconception on my part.

I am aware that with some frequency a stroke patient suffers a severe denial of disability associated with his illness or of some residual defect. As I learned, the term *anosognosia* is generally used to refer to an unawareness of some aspect of a disease process, including even a complete denial of a hemiplegia. There is as yet no general agreement concerning the etiology and significance of this defense. It seems that it is not so much the site or even the side of the lesion as much as it is a common and even characteristic feature of cerebral disease in general, and that certain types of personality traits existing before the neurological damage may well play some part in determining the patient's attitude toward his disability (Ullman, 1962). I have sometimes thought that in terms of my reaction toward the remaining deficits I would be better off if I could summon some denial rather than always being supersensitive to the residual manifestations of my disability, but apparently one doesn't have a choice in this matter.

Despite my emphasis on pathology, I like to believe that I appear to have remained largely the same person that I was before. I have no difficulty in physical or motor activities (outside of typing or especially writing) and no perceptual disturbances, and I think my judgment is unimpaired. Even the first morning when I awoke aphasic, my wife said clever little things to me and I attempted to respond with a smile (Bette told me later that it was a one-sided smile since the paralysis did not leave my face for several days). The main effect of the stroke on my personality has been twofold: generally, as I have mentioned, I have the tendency to withdraw or avoid most social contacts; and specifically, aphasia has played hob with my humor since I can no longer make spontaneous remarks with the superb sense of timing that I am sure I previously displayed!

During the summer term in 1968 I helped assess potential clients to be seen by students in the fall at the clinic. This was one of the first times that I felt exposed, since there is absolutely no way to plan for the highly individualistic problems presented to me. However, I drew upon my years of diagnostic experience and only occasionally goofed, e.g., once I persistently called a young child Kevin when his name was Scott; his parents were so overawed by the formalities that they never corrected me and I only caught it when I listened to the tape. Considering everything, I felt that I did an adequate job in interviewing and wrote some reasonably good diagnostic reports.

In the fall I continued to teach a psychotherapy laboratory and also began instruction in a course designed to teach students an awareness of the hypnosymbolic use of dreams and fantasy. In this course I attempted a change of pace from my former teaching technique, giving a didactic lecture during the first hour, followed by the playing of relevant tapes illustrative of the points that I had stressed. It occurred to me later that my very first dream after the cerebral insult was predictive of the way that I structured the course.

I still have real difficulty in composing and delivering my lectures. I tend to compensate by writing them down in complete and highly exact detail before delivering a lecture. I continue to tell myself that I can write or lecture or conduct research — it is only that it takes longer. I guess I haven't resigned myself yet to the fact that I am no longer as verbally fluent as I was earlier. This is a tremendous step for a person who throughout his lifetime could count on his ability to persuade others to his point of view and in effect sell his ideas through his ability to communicate.

Although I have undergone numerous diagnostic procedures we really have no real knowledge of either the precipitating or the predisposing factors in my illness. The experts vaguely refer to the fact that perhaps at some time earlier — even twenty years ago — I sustained damage to the artery which became apparent when I suffered my stroke. The physicians will not admit that my cold had anything whatsoever to do with my stroke, and I am about ready to agree with them. Probably the hard cough which I suffered for the two weeks before my accident was really due to the fact that the artery was being slowly closed; at the moment of the stroke the cough completely disappeared, and rather surprisingly I haven't had a cold since. The single period that I had been hospitalized earlier was when I spent a part of a month in a military hospital for a combination of a left mastoid infection, a tonsillectomy, and measles. At that time, for the one and only period in my life, I suffered excruciating head-aches. When discharged from the service at the age of twenty-one, I applied for a disability allowance due to the fact that I was prone to develop episodes involving a very painful and stiff neck, but it was disallowed. I continued to experience this stiffness periodically for eight to ten years, but it gradually disappeared.

I have maintained that I had no premorbid symptoms, which is technically true, but two years before we left San Francisco I was bothered by two temporary yet troublesome afflictions. I began developing leg cramps while sleeping. When I happened to complain of this development, the regional mental health director spoke knowingly, and said that it was probably due to my growing older, since he had experienced the same condition for some years. It may be of some significance that I suffered no cramps once I came to the university.

A year before we left, I took charge of the mental health program in the western region when the associate mental health director took leave for six months to conduct a tour of mental health conditions in the new and developing countries of Africa and Asia. During this period my other symptom developed. It was more serious and prompted me to seek the medical advice of an internist (i.e., "Uncle George"). For several months, usually immediately after lunch, I would develop a condition where the periphery of both eyes was surrounded by an aura of bright color and I would find "holes" in my field of vision, about where I imagined the nerve would enter the back of the retina. After a series of tests the internist came to the conclusion that possibly I was a borderline diabetic. He prescribed a diet for me which I held to for a couple of months. In thinking back, this may have been the first neurophysiological sign of the coming stroke. The condition cleared up over time and I promptly forgot about it.

Let me also mention, while I am on the matter, two other potential health hazards. Even before graduation from high school my weight fluctuated by fifteen to twenty pounds yearly. I tended to gain in the winter and take it off in the spring. As time and age mounted, I found it increasingly more difficult to shed the weight each year and was overweight by twenty-five pounds at the time of the stroke. The other thing has to do with a peculiar condition of my veins and arteries. In tenth grade I volunteered to give blood for a classmate who had leukemia. The doctor had to puncture six or seven veins *in each arm* because the veins would collapse and the flow of blood would stop. I had forged my mother's signature to the permission slip; later she was shocked when I assisted her in hanging up some wet clothes and I inadvertently revealed my coal black arms. Who knows whether any or all or none of these were related to my cerebral accident.

About four months after the stroke, I began laboriously to keep notes on my condition, and now I have begun writing an account of my personal experience for possible journal publication, basically for three reasons. First, because this is a unique experience for anyone of my age and particular professional background to suffer, and I am sufficiently pleased about my recovery and compulsive enough to want to document it; second, for whatever insights this record may contribute to professional people who have an interest in gaining knowledge of cerebral pathology and what they might do to partially alleviate it; and third, to attempt to give some understanding to my friends and colleagues who often, in their contact with me, maintain, to me at least, that they do not have the perception of any dramatic deficiency in my speech and writing.

This experience is a lonely one for an aphasic and his family. Even though I am at a major university and a member of an outstanding psychology department, I have reluctantly come to the conclusion that no one really knows much about how to treat my brand of aphasia. We have conferred with a number of authorities and all of them say that this sort of thing takes time and they can do nothing specifically to assist me. Joe Wepman is doubtlessly correct when he estimates that only 30 percent of aphasics get treated (Jones & Wepman, 1964). There are, of course, numerous treatment centers for patients who have suffered massive strokes and attempts are made in physical therapy for their gross deficiences. My residual disability isn't with speech per se, but rather is with a disorganization in the brain which gives rise to difficulties primarily in word-finding signs or what some experts have termed *nominal aphasia*. I have maintained that my residual disability is no more than 10 percent — I simply fail to recall highly significant and special words that I would like to use. I know what I want to say, but cannot get at the words at that particular moment. This is a problem in selecting the precise informational words needed to communicate my thoughts accurately in either external communication or even internal speech.

There are two alternative explanations for this situation: I possess an organic deficit with an overlay of anxiety or I suffer a basic lack of self-confidence due to my accident, with some residual organic component. It is more hopeful for me to stress the second alternative — it leaves me something that I can continue to work on. My progress will in part be affected by the continued tolerance of my colleagues and the good will of my speech therapist, but in large measure my further recovery from my disability will eventually come about through the passage of time, through continued hard work with my wife, and through remaining highly motivated and not becoming too discouraged to continue working on the problem.

While I have not been overly preoccupied with thoughts of self-destruction, the idea of suicide does occasionally cross my mind. I am reminded that almost twenty-five years ago I attended a course given by Professor Harry Harlow in physiological psychology. He was a compulsive, though witty and sometimes cynical, teacher. I recall the essence of a story which he told, to wit, that God had made the porpoise in a fit of malicious wrath. Next to man and the apes, the porpoise supposedly had the highest intelligence of any mammal, but it had been given no mechanism for expressing its creative thoughts.

Harlow maintained that he could think of nothing more damaging to the ego than to have an intelligent brain but no equipment for expressing it. Nor can I.

References

Jones, L. V., and Wepman, J. M. 1965. Aphasia research opens new insights into brain mechanisms. In *Research Project Summaries* (No. 2), Bethesda: NIMH, pp. 69-77.

Ullman, M. 1962. *Behavioral changes in patients following strokes.* Springfield, Ill.: C. C. Thomas, pp. 69-93.

4

Speech Therapy

WITH ROBERT K. SIMPSON

I

SIMPSON: Scott Moss first came to the Speech and Hearing Clinic of the University of Illinois on January 26, 1968. This was approximately three months after his CVA. At that time he was functioning at a rather high level when compared to most aphasics. However, when compared with his pre-traumatic level there were certainly areas of deficiency. As examples, during the Schuell Short Examination for Aphasia, Dr. Moss was able to repeat only nine of the ten sentences correctly. He missed two of the six questions concerning an orally presented paragraph and one of five questions on the paragraph, which he read silently. His definition of island was "surrounded by water" and his definition of motor was "make car go." His explanation of the proverb "Don't change horses in the middle of a stream" was "don't attempt to — don't change horses or whatever body in — in the midst of strife." He had three errors in reproducing symbols and missed one out of six sentences in writing from dictation. The Peabody Picture Vocabulary Test was also administered. Although this test was not designed to be used with adult aphasics, it is sometimes helpful in giving an indication of receptive vocabulary. Dr. Moss's performance was less than acceptable for the average eighteen-year-old.[1]

[1] I was surprised when I read this, that is, the errors that I had made. When

The test results were summarized rather well by the examiner:

Dr. Moss presents a rather complicated picture since damage is minimal as compared to most aphasics but definitely a problem to the person in question. . . . Even though very little impairment of communicative abilities was evident in general conversation, it was apparent to the examiner that Dr. Moss was performing at a lower level than one would expect of a person with his training and reported facility with language. . . . Prognosis for near normal communication is good, if one looks at test results as measured by the Schuell Examination. The question which remains in view of test results is, will a person of Dr. Moss's pre-trauma state be willing to accept less than this and how much of recovery of the pre-trauma state will be difficult to attain without help to allay some of the psychological and intellectual fears which may very well inhibit language training.

Therapy was initiated on February 12, 1968. During this initial therapy it was possible to delineate Dr. Moss's specific problems in more detail. First, he had difficulty in recalling specific words which were part of his professional vocabulary. In general social conversation this difficulty was not readily evident, for when he could not find one word he could rapidly substitute another for it. When the requirements of professional language necessitated a specific word which could not easily be substituted, he had difficulty. Second, he had a problem in retention. This retention problem was demonstrated on the input side by his difficulty in retaining one thought long enough to relate it to a second thought. This was also demonstrated in the output by his difficulty in retaining a thought long enough to allow an appropriate verbal response. Dr. Moss often talked about his problem in "organizing his thoughts" and the reduced transient memory was one of the main contributing factors to this problem in organization. Third, he did not like to admit openly that he had problems in communication. This is certainly an understandable attitude and does have both positive and negative features. On the positive side, this

---

I made the original contact with the speech clinic staff member, I was requested to come to a rather elegant new nursing home and found that she had set up a testing situation before the nursing staff. Fortunately this situation did not cause any considerable increase in anxiety as I recall, and I came away elated at my performance, since this was my first "social contact" since my stroke. Still, there was some self-deception (anosognosia). *C.S.M.*

provided a great deal of motivation to improve to the extent that no one would ever know that he had a problem. On the negative side, it kept him from benefiting from one excellent source of stimulation: interaction with his colleagues on a professional level.

When these problems became evident, the general plan of therapy then became apparent. Some type of therapy was needed to enable him to recall the professional terms more quickly and accurately. Some type of therapy was needed to help him improve his transient memory. And some type of therapy was needed to alter his attitude or at least his practices so that he could benefit from the stimulation of interchange with his professional colleagues. Although there was some direct drill on definitions, much of the therapy was designed to incorporate both practice in word-finding and procedures to increase his retention span. One of the more productive techniques or activities was having Dr. Moss read and outline a paragraph from a professional article. He then related the information included in the paragraph, first with the aid of the outline and then without it. Following this he would write from memory the basic ideas of the paragraph. The length of these assignments was gradually increased from single paragraphs to complete articles.

As can be seen, Dr. Moss was already in transition between stage one and stage two in speech therapy; that is, he was already proceeding from formal, uniform exercises given most aphasics in the clinic to practices assigned to resolve his unique problems. There were some specific drills and exercises which could be presented in a more formal and traditional approach. However, most of his needs were unique to him and therefore he had to assume much of the responsibility for determining these needs and directing therapy. The best therapy for him at this point consisted of the activities of his daily living. These gave him the most appropriate stimulation and the best chance to utilize and practice his abilities. In the areas of social interaction there was no problem, for he was assuming a near-normal social life. In the professional area there was a problem, for he had a great fear of showing his temporary inadequacies to either his colleagues or students and restricted his interaction as much as possible. However, he was involved in a professional activity which tended to counter-balance this deficiency. With the help of his wife he continued to write five articles which he had planned (and had made a commitment to himself) to write prior to the CVA. This was a difficult task and one which the therapist certainly would not have assigned. However, it was very beneficial, for it did give him the stimulation of professional language, which he needed, and provided this stimulation in the secure environment of his own home. He could demonstrate his inadequacies to his wife without unduly increasing his level of anxiety. Undoubtedly, his wife was his best therapist.

Dr. Moss was scheduled to teach another class during the fall semester of 1968, "Community Psychology." This assignment did cause some fear and doubts concerning his capabilities. Therefore, during the preceding summer the main objective of therapy was to demonstrate to him that he could be quite successful. To do this Dr. Moss outlined prepared lectures which he would use in the fall. These were presented to the therapist with the therapist acting as a student. At first the lectures were presented in the optimal environment. As he became more secure the therapist reacted as a student by (1) interrupting the lecture to ask questions; (2) requiring Dr. Moss to explain in a different way or elaborate on a certain point; (3) performing distractions, such as not attending to the lecture and asking him to repeat what he had previously discussed because the therapist had not been paying attention; (4) allowing environmental sounds or other people to interrupt the lecture and asking Dr. Moss to continue. We were trying to build up his confidence and his tolerance for ambiguity and unstructuredness.

II

Moss: Segments of three consecutive sessions, taken in February, 1969, depict the typical sequence of events that constituted formal treatment at still a later stage of speech therapy. They indicate how I still fluctuated sixteen months after the accident, depending on my general state of health at the moment, the degree of tiredness which I experienced, and, primarily, who I was relating to and what I was called upon to do. Specifically, I interpreted these sessions as showing a progressive lessening of self-sufficiency in the areas tested, ranging from relative competence in the area of visual and audio retention, through the handling of synonyms, to a decidedly shaky dealing with definitions of professional terminology. The last session, in particular, represents the type of situation that I tended to avoid whenever possible, that is, where the attention was focused on me in an open-ended situation, in the expectation that I would conceptualize and at the same time provide the words, and where the set was constantly shifted.

February 1, 1969

Moss: I'm teaching a course in community mental health and I'm trying to give the students a variety of experiences and I accomplish this in different ways. For example, through the texts, through various brochures, each two-hour session I devote one hour to having someone come in and tell about their experience in community mental health, and then I've divided them into groups and each of them are taking the local mental health services to various populations. They have the responsibility of actually conducting a session on their particular topics about twelve weeks from now. They actually go out into the community and familiarize themselves with the programs in the community and then will undertake to represent it to the other students, where the community is at in services to the particular population, what is good and what is bad about it, and then make recommendations in terms of what they have been taught primarily from behavior theory. This sort of brings it home to them.

Ther.: Last semester you had a practicum and what else, a seminar?

Moss: Yes, hypnotherapy.

Ther.: And how many were in those?

Moss: About eight and eight.

Ther.: Is this the biggest class you had?

Moss: Yes, and it's the first formal class as well, where I have to get up and lecture.

Ther.: Graduate students? Did you say anything to them, and I don't think you will really have to, about the stroke and the fact that there might be some language impairment apparent?

Moss: I did tell them last semester, I didn't tell them this semester. I assume that some students may know this, but other students may not, but I feel at this stage I should compensate for any deficiencies I have, and my experience last year was that most of the questions that they brought up, I found that I could answer them. So I really didn't stumble about very much. I think the answers I gave were relatively short answers. They were not the way I might have expounded on a subject at one time, because I still find more difficulty in organizing my thoughts than I did formerly. Whereas before I could answer most any question automatically, now it takes me some time to think through and put them in a language that the students can comprehend.

THER.: Do you use class notes? How much do you rely on them?

Moss: Yes, and I rely on them a great deal.

THER.: Is that like reading from them, to some extent; just a glance down to see where you are, or what?

Moss: I think I described to you the elaborate ritual that I must go through before each class. I try to anticipate all possible questions and frame the answers to them, and the notes that I have are complete in unusual detail. I am quite aware this isn't the way you treat — teach graduate students, so that I attempt to put on an act and appear more casual about my notes than I actually am. But I find that I have to glance down at my notes very frequently because otherwise, if I don't do this, I tend to get lost in what I am saying. I'll make a point and if I don't refer back to my notes at that juncture I will hesitate, and once I hesitate then I'll block, and once I block then I have a very difficult time. That's more or less what I do.

THER.: Let me check in your folder, and look at your last test. A woman named Hildred Schuell developed a test for aphasia, but it is not sensitive enough to pick up impairment for someone like you. I don't think there is anything on it.

Moss: Is this the test that I took for Mrs. Arlt?

THER.: It might have been the shorter version. I think there is only one thing I'd like to have you do — check out your writing ability. I think we have a sample from September which might give us some comparison.

Moss: I don't think it's changed much.

THER.: I don't know. The impression is that you're more fluent now. You have five minutes to look at a picture and write what you can about it in the next five minutes. Do you have a pencil?

Moss: Shall I write it out in narrative form or is it all right —

Ther.: Let me read the instructions to you. "Write a paragraph about this picture, about what is happening. Write as much as you can." O.K.?

[I viewed the picture and then wrote down what I remembered, namely, it was a rustic scene composed of members of a family engaged in various pursuits in the yard of their home.]

Ther.: How is your writing?

Moss: That's my best effort.

Ther.: It seems like last semester you supposedly became able to write for a longer period of time without having your writing become less readable.

Moss: I definitely try to keep myself under control and not let it happen this time.

Ther.: It looks like you have maintained the same degree of control this time.

Moss: Yes, although it's difficult, before I would have let go. But I have become fairly more accomplished in my typing.

Ther.: You have? Are you doing a lot of typing at home because you have to?

Moss: Yes, but where formerly I would have typed fifty to sixty words per minute, now I can type maybe half that much, with many more errors — and yet I am always aware of when these errors occur.

Ther.: I'm going to read you an article and after I've finished reading it, I'll ask you some questions about it. It's going to be lengthy but I don't think it's going to be so lengthy that it will make that much difference. This is on smoking, "The Strickman Filter."

"After eight years of working at home, in his home laboratory, Strickman, a New Jersey chemist claimed the grand prize in cigarette research, a filter which removed two-thirds of the tar and nicotine, and unlike other filters, it does not destroy the tobacco taste. Robert L. Strickman, fifty-six, had impressive background for his discovery. With full fanfare, it was announced by Columbia University President, Grayson Kirk, and Dr. H. Houston Merritt, dean of Columbia's College of Physicians and Surgeons, that Strickman gave full rights to the filter to the university, a gift which may well bring the university millions in licensing fees. Strickman remains tightlipped about how his filter works, unwilling to jeopardize his pending patent; he merely says his filter consists of a new type of crystalline, nontoxic polymer that works by selective trapping, perhaps based on ion exchange in electrostatic action. He claims it costs little to produce and can be part of the cigarette or used in cigarette holders."

O.K. Generally, what have I said?

Moss: Well, it's about this man's invention, Strickman. He invented an improved cigarette filter, and apparently he has associated himself with Columbia University and this is a press conference that was held to announce this filter to the public.

THER.: What's his occupation or profession?

Moss: Chemist?

THER.: Do you remember where he's from?

Moss: Some place in New Jersey, I don't remember the city.

THER.: What does his filter do that supposedly other filters haven't done so far?

Moss: It does two things. It filters a great deal more of tar and other things, nicotine, supposedly it filters out two-thirds more than other filters, and it also preserves the flavor.

THER.: Do you remember how old he was?

Moss: Oh dear. I don't know, I'll guess he's fifty-two. (Ther. volunteers age fifty-six.) I don't remember who the president of the university is or the name of the dean of the medical school.

THER.: Do you remember what he said his filter consists of?

Moss: Not really. He used a term which implies to me it was made up of — it sounded like, and this isn't it, but it's somewhat like it, polymere? I don't remember the rest of it but it had the connotation of some sort of a synthetic filter which had the properties of somehow transporting or exchanging the ions, but more than that I can't tell you.

THER.: He named another advantage, one of the last things I said.

Moss: It would have to be, of course, very economical to produce.

THER.: Excellent! I don't think you have missed any of the information that is in here. Something has happened with this case, have you heard about it in the news?

Moss: They apparently made this pronouncement but it didn't work out the way they had claimed and Columbia was in the process of withdrawing their sponsorship. But what specifically it was, I don't know. I'm not sure the public was informed as to what the problem was, but it is interesting that this would happen because by the time they got around to this pronouncement, it had been tested repeatedly in the laboratory.

Ther.: Well, I have the impression it wasn't working the way they said it would.

Moss: And this meant that perhaps Columbia University wasn't a participant in the earlier laboratory work on the filter.

Ther.: Now I want you to read from here down to here, and I'll ask you questions about it.

[Twenty-seven-second pause]

Ther.: Have you finished reading it?

Moss: Yes, more or less. I'm just trying to figure how it works [in looking at a diagram].

Ther.: This is really a topic of discussion now. It's on every discussion program, preventing air collisions.

Moss: I'm not really sure I understand the relationship between the aircraft and the ground mechanism.

Ther.: How about your telling me everything you did understand?

Moss: Well, let's see. The airlines and the federal government are attempting to concoct some sort of a collision-avoidance system. This is necessary because they estimate 400 near misses occur each year and it will grow worse with more planes in the air, plus the fact that we'll have supersonic transports and jumbo transports. So they can't avoid this question much longer. They think they have an answer, in that their plan is to equip each transport with an atomic clock and a computer. This they can do for approximately $40,000 per plane. Now I'm kind of vague on this, but one way or another the plane will be enveloped in an electronic field, somehow the electronic timer on these planes has a relationship to the ground, this is because the time of these planes must be absolutely the same; whenever possible they have a master clock on the ground which within a certain radius gears in all the clocks. Supposedly when two bubbles converge, this will set off a warning system, supposedly it's an audio-visual warning system, in addition it may give the pilot a mild shock, but somehow or other it will alert him to the impending danger of a collision. These bubbles of two converging planes will intersperse at a distance of, in time, one minute, and at a distance of 20 miles apart. And this will trigger off the computer and a short distance later — 20 seconds? — the computer will tell the pilot which way to move the aircraft in order to avoid the collision. Where it isn't possible to have the coordinating ground facilities in relation to the different clocks in the airplanes then supposedly they'll have an arrangement whereby the timing device in one aircraft assumes the master control of all aircrafts in the vicinity and will quickly adjust the other clocks in the other aircrafts to hone in on its own.

THER.: All that I have left are some very trivial questions: What is the CAS that they refer to in the article?

MOSS: Collision-Avoidance System, I suppose.

THER.: And ATA is —

MOSS: [Pause]

THER.: The Air Transport Association.

MOSS: Right, I couldn't figure what the final A was.

THER.: When do they hope to have this in operation?

MOSS: That's a good question, I suppose it is in the last lines in the article. I don't know. My hunch is that this is something that is feasible but they haven't yet got around to saying when it will actually go into operation. Now what does it really say?

THER.: They hope to have it in operation by 1971. They supposedly have a prototype that is actually being refined. Again such minor things. We have norms for what a person should get but there isn't any type of test material advanced enough to rate you on, but judging from this you have very little problem.

MOSS: Using my own norms I would say that I comprehend this — I comprehend most of what I read now — but it takes more time than before.[2] It is difficult to say what the matter is but in a way it is somewhat similar to my writing. When I am not writing for someone my handwriting tends to scrawl off; I think it is something like this

---

[2] I was very pleased that I had come through this session so well and to find that my immediate memory was intact.

in reading and writing and talking that it is difficult to keep a governor on. Now I am definitely pacing myself to spell out my communications to you but it would be relatively easy to let my speech deteriorate the same as my handwriting.

THER.: By deteriorate, how do you mean? Are you now constantly looking for words?

Moss: It isn't as bad as it was six months ago — more words come to me automatically. One thing that I have found out in the last few months, I have taped a number of my sessions and I was really amazed to find that for the most part my speech went well.

THER.: You were amazed?! [she sounds incredulous]

Moss: Because if you ask me how the speech goes I am so caught up in trying to formulate the speech I no longer pay much attention to how it comes out. A normal person, like yourself — or as I was — part of you attends to what you are saying — ah — now I still attend to what I am saying and for the most part would catch myself if I made a gross error, but much more of my attention is focused inwardly trying to select the proper words.

THER.: Of course, the most emphasis in normal speech is on what you are saying.

Moss: Right, but not how you say it —

THER.: There is more emphasis on *how* you are saying it?

Moss: Very much so, so this is an explanation of my amazement —

THER.: You mean *how* you are putting words together —

Moss: Selecting words.

THER.: I mean the motor act of saying certain sounds, but you've never had trouble in saying sounds —

Moss: At least not when I became fluent again.

THER.: Now you say that you must attend much more to how you are speaking, what does this mean?

Moss: I still haven't got across the point I want to make. Do you mind if I pace, it makes it easier.[3] What I am trying to get across is that before the accident I was like most people, I attended to what

---

[3] During this period I often strolled back and forth in my conversations with people: the peripatetics served to use some of the undifferentiated energy that was released while I struggled to find words to put them into sentences. It is perhaps an exaggeration of the foot tapping that many anxious but normal people engage in.

I was saying; now my attention is deflected into trying to find the right words. This is something that the ordinary person doesn't bother with so that much of my attention is focused on conjuring up words that I am going to say. And this makes me so anxious that when I listened to myself on the tapes I was amazed to find that none of this got through. When I listened to the tapes there were two normal people engaged in conversation.

THER.: And this is what other people hear.

MOSS: But my anxiety over the production of words is so great that I thought automatically that it interfered with my speech as well.

THER.: That is very interesting, because even though you were telling me about your problem, I heard only minimal difficulties. I felt there were more anxieties but I couldn't crawl inside of you —

MOSS: I accept the fact that I am now about as fluent as I ever was. But then comes the question — why do I still feel as anxious in communicating with others and I have tried to explain what I think it is due to. The anxiety over being able to reach into your mind and pick out the appropriate words and be able to string them together. It is a focus on this process, whereas before it was a focus on how you said things, not the selection of what you said.

THER.: Before you said things and the words just flowed, now you have the idea but have to find the words to express it.

MOSS: It is a very great — trauma to be in constant interaction with another person when you are not aware of where the next word will come from and this is what I am worried about. You have no idea as to how much stress goes into my production of the speech that I deliver to you now. It is a little bit like Fairbanks' Delayed Feedback machine that causes stuttering in normal persons — this is how I feel every time that I get into communication with another person.

February 17, 1969

THER.: Are you having trouble with your speech, more, less, the same?

MOSS: It is very much leveled off. I really don't detect I have any trouble with my speech unless I become anxious, but this is because I still steer away from exposing myself to anyone unless it is absolutely necessary. In other words, what I am really saying is I am

now neither progressing nor regressing, except for specific instances
where I perhaps am more anxious than otherwise and then I will
have difficulty.

THER.: The reason I asked was that you read that [a summary of a
preceding reprint of mine which I had brought into the therapist],
and I wanted you just to tell me. Have you done a lot of that?

Moss: Yes, certainly, as much as possible —

THER.: Because you don't have to reveal your limitations? I can
understand that.

Moss: To actually get up in front of a class and conduct a lecture
is exceedingly difficult for me, so I go through a great — I want to
say vogue, but that's not it — I go through the vogue of trying to
anticipate all possible questions that can come up. I put them down
so that I have them in front of me. But for the most part I stick
very closely to the notes, without attemping to give the appearance
of reading them. But it must be apparent too that I am doing this,
to some of the students at least.

THER.: Has anyone said anything about it? Have they given that
indication?

Moss: Not directly, no.

THER.: Do you think that they're not gaining as much from your
lectures?

Moss: Oh, yes. Before the accident I was more or less literal when
subjects were brought up, but now when they bring up subjects
that I don't anticipate or haven't prepared an answer on paper, this
throws me, do you see? And I really can't answer it very well, because I would really expose the fact that I have a decided verbal —
I have a decided verbal —

THER.: Decrease in your verbal ability?

Moss: That's fine.

THER.: Why haven't you told the class? I think you should.

Moss: I debated about this. I did it last semester and things went
relatively swimmingly, largely because of the way I structured the
course. At least half of each session was taken by playing over tapes
that I had done previously and then I engaged in a question-answer
relationship. There I could conduct myself relatively easily, with
emphasis on *relatively*. But to get up in front of a class and to talk

for two hours is quite another thing, you see. There the limitation that I talked about will become most apparent if I deviate much from the notes. So anyway, I haven't told the class this semester, although I am sure that many of the students know about my accident.

THER.: Have you given any more consideration to taking another job?

MOSS: Yes, certainly, I live by this day by day, trying to take on the responsibility of class and so on, and always in the back of my mind is perhaps taking some job and leaving go of this one. But it is a hard thing to do for a couple of reasons. For one thing I still have the ambition to train graduate students; this is what I wanted to do when I came here and I'm struggling against what happened, trying to attain something like what I would have done if I hadn't had the accident. I haven't really entirely given up on my objective.

THER.: I'd be disappointed in you if you did.

MOSS: The second thing which deters me from looking at other positions is that I have no confidence that I can go into another position and represent myself the way I would have formerly. So those two things in combination make it very difficult to consider another position at this time.

THER.: I understand. Do you have any more unusual trouble thinking of words?

MOSS: Not any more trouble than I had four or five months ago.

THER.: Let's try something that we tried last semester. Let's try some synonyms again. These are easy words, but let's begin with them: business. It's a word that you use every day but you don't actually think about it.

MOSS: Ah, work, profession, daily tasks, routine —

THER.: How about occupation. Daily tasks is a good one because it is general.

MOSS: Naturally it is very easy to give a number of examples but I'm trying not to do that.

THER.: Good. I don't want you to do that.

MOSS: Let's see if I can think of any others. I suppose you could use the term avocation.

THER.: Can you define business?

MOSS: A type of work that one gets paid for.

THER.: The type of work one does rather than the work that one gets paid for, since sometimes you aren't paid for it.

Moss: If you aren't paid it probably wouldn't fit the definition of work.

THER.: Let's try negotiate, A synonym first.

Moss: Something like barter. Negotiate — now I'm blocking. Rather than just barter I don't know — ah —

THER.: Confer? But there's more to it than confer —

Moss: You have to arrive at some agreement. Entering into a conference is the beginning of negotiating.

THER.: To negotiate is to confer. The dictionary says it is "to deal or manage, to arrange for." Liberal? [At that juncture I begin to pace.] Does it help you not to block to walk around?

Moss : It's a way of expending energy. I've found that it helps. Some who hold to different points of view —

THER.: What do you think is a general definition of liberal? How about free — is that appropriate? What is the antonym?

Moss: Conservative. A Democrat versus a Republican. It is someone that is open to new ideas.

THER.: That's right. Generous, even.

Moss: I wouldn't have considered that — possibly.

THER.: Broadminded, tolerant —

Moss: Although in terms of liberals today many of them are anti-tolerant. I'm not sure that holds anymore, at least in the way we are experiencing it. It's a question of where you stand when you make this evaluation.

THER.: That's an interesting point that you brought up. How about response?

Moss: Reaction.

THER.: Good. Here's a real easy one: To respond is to — [pause]

Moss: You've got me.

THER.: Answer.

Moss: Yes, I didn't think of that. I think the reason I didn't is that it is a very concrete form of response and that would cause a shift in my set. I wonder how much of this is due to the fact of establishing a set?

THER.: Do you have difficulty in this or is it because you are here and working so hard to be correct in all of your answers and to do well — that's anxiety-producing in itself.

Moss: But this may be a general factor. Perhaps I am wrong but it seems that I have difficulty in shifting sets. This is reflected in the types of questions that graduate students ask me. I attempt to anticipate the questions, but if I haven't anticipated a line of questioning that will ensue then I am very much at a loss to shift over to what they are talking about and to make any sense at all out of it. If they give me time to stop and think about what they are saying then I can as likely as not come up with a reasonable answer, but this may be a part of the difficulty that I suffer from — just of the fluidity, the flexibility of being *liberal* in shifting from one set to another. I think that when people shift sets on me this arouses anxiety which results in my blocking on anything that they are talking about.

Ther.: Anxiety will do that in any case.

Moss: Yes, but again I'm commenting on a relative thing. Two years ago I wouldn't have had the same experience.

Ther.: Can you think of another answer to "respond"?

Moss: Again it is characteristic when you ask a question like this I will usually be able to respond with something appropriate, but only one or two things.[4] I think this gets nearer the cause of some of my disability than practically anything else we do. For example, at an earlier time, you read paragraphs and had me — testing my ability to —

Ther.: Auditory retention?

Moss: Gee, I never would have come up with that. Auditory retention. For the most part I don't think I suffer much of a disability in this area, but this in-depth sort of a thing is designed for a person who has aphasia, you read it or I read it, and then it is easy to retain for the moment. I have much more difficulty in — I've got to be careful here — that's not correct what I was going to say — and if I answer you in terms of specific questions it is relatively easy, even if you ask the question generally, "What was the article about?," I can remember enough so that I have to — what I have

⁴ Contrast this to my statements made right after the stroke that when I would block absolutely no associations would present themselves to my mind (p. 9).

to say into anything like a context with which you present a lecture. So it is relatively easy to tell you what the article was about, because I — let me stop —

THER.: Let me ask you a question while you are stuck. Do you talk about your disabilities like this to anyone else? Or as frequently as you do to me?

Moss: No, not other than my wife. I bend her ear frequently about the difficulties I am having and what they are like. Possibly the other person is a new addition to the clinical faculty who is in consulting — community — mental health. We have two meetings a week and it is apparent in our interchange that I am having difficulty so I'll frequently stop and comment about what the problems seem to be. Other than those instances I don't comment to anyone about it. This makes quite a problem because there are many issues that are brought up which I should discuss with other members of the faculty — for example, I am now on a committee for screening admissions. I thought I had this all worked out until it became apparent to me that they wanted me to take on additional duties which I knew nothing about. At that point I could have gone around to the other faculty members and asked them about this new problem — it has to do with research and teaching assistantships to the graduate school for the clinical psychology department — but when I approach other faculty members this poses a great problem. Because while I know generally what I want to talk to them about, just to go in and start a conversation with them it is fraught with anxiety because in the middle of a sentence I may simply block — and what do you do then?

THER.: That's why I think you are wrong by not telling them that you do have the disability. It will only result in harm. Say you do block with fellow workers — the fear mounts and you wonder what is going through their minds at the same time. This shows that Dr. Moss has limitations. Whereas if you explained this, the anxiety would be greatly reduced for you. When you have a block here, with me, it's not the fact that I'm thinking that you have limitations, it is of the block itself, it doesn't lower you in my estimation. It doesn't make me feel that you don't know your field. In contrast, I think you would have this feeling for people who don't know.

Moss: The thing which gives me freedom to block to you is because
I have entered into a patient-therapist relationship, do you see?
This is entirely different once you have attempted to relate to a
peer group, to colleagues.

Ther.: Yes, I can understand and I realize what you mean, but I
still think that this would reduce a lot of anxiety.

Moss: You may be correct —

Ther.: Did you ever have this feeling, that you felt more comfortable
with someone who knew of your stroke?

Moss: I feel much more comfortable with the person that I alluded to
a moment ago, because he knows and I have no pretense — if I block
I block and I simply stumble about until I unblock. It is much more
comfortable but I couldn't for a moment attempt this with a class,
because the give and take that we engage in in our private sessions
is not conducted at the abstract level the class is held in. Much of
the verbalization between us doesn't have to be highly explicit —
we understand what each other means — we are talking about
things that the other already knows. The role of the teacher I don't
see as being commensurate with the role of the patient, do you see?

Ther.: I do see what you mean but I also mean that you should see
my point, too. In the role of teacher you are bringing them up to
your level, but also you don't want them to know that there are
limitations on your level.

Moss: Say it again — say it another way.

Ther.: Yes, Doctor — you feel maybe that there would be a loss of
esteem if they knew of these limitations, but if they knew there was a
reason for you to have these limitations, I don't think there would
be any loss of esteem.

Moss: I think there would be, but they would have a ready rationalization in terms of this accident. They can look on it, hopefully,
as a clinician would, but this gives rise then to many questions as
to whether I should continue to teach. Of course, that question is
always in my mind. How far one goes in attempting to compensate
for a limitation, particularly this limitation. Actually, perhaps I
would do better to get out of this position because certainly most
other jobs would not be as anxiety-filled as this one. But at this
juncture I have obtained a stature that whenever anybody thinks of

me for a job one question which comes before their mind is trying to find a job which is conceptually big enough, there would be enough money, etc., that I would be attracted to it. The people I have made preliminary contacts with have always had in mind for — for what? for what? —

THER.: If I knew I would tell you.

MOSS: That would call for a highly elevated individual. This is another dilemma that I'm in because the jobs that could become available to me are pitched at a level of what I could have accomplished before the accident. When I try to explain to these people that I have all sorts of reservations about taking a job like this, they don't believe it.

THER.: You don't think you can function on the same level — that these jobs would be too much for you, that you could not achieve that level again?

MOSS: You're correct in my appraisal of the fact that I could not do it. So this is another limiting factor in searching out any other position. Actually, I have thought many times recently that I would be happy reverting into a clinician again, perhaps having charge of a group of patients or a ward. I think that at least I can begin there — I would feel comfortable in that type of responsibility.

February 24, 1970

MOSS: I'm tired. I've just finished with my community mental health session, and following that, I had a subcommittee meeting which took me almost to 4:00. I've divided the students into three groups and they're attempting to learn what the local agencies do in reference with the aged, children, and the disadvantaged. So I meet with one of those committees after the class session. By this time I'm done [in].

THER.: You said you were teaching them about hospitals, are you going to hospitals in this area?

MOSS: I don't really remember telling you that I was teaching them about hospitals — community mental health is the — opposite of hospitals. But they will have some contact with hospitals. For example, they will meet with Dr. Rohlke, Roffes, Rothes, who is the head psychiatrist over at Mercy — the fifth floor unit, the psychiatric unit. But this may be as much contact as they have with the hospital.

THER.: They use the term "chronic brain syndrome" in hospitals — how do you define it?

MOSS: I think it is often the diagnosis that is given in lieu of finding anything specific about the person. They simply test the person who is middle aged or older and he tests erratic on different intelligence tests and so on that they give —

THER.: What do you mean by erratic?

MOSS: Well, for example, on the Weschler-Bellevue where they have different scales which attempt to measure something specific about intelligence and they aren't highly intercorrelated to any degree. He will often be too high on one thing and below on another thing. Now this does happen even with the best of people because as you get older you tend to specialize, but let's say he has an abnormal — now what's the word for it — amount of variance on these scales. That plus the fact that many of these people are — (longer pause) — are a — socially sort of burnt out.[5]

THER.: How else would you say that?

MOSS: I thought it was a good term (laughs). They don't tend to be — they tend to react highly selectively to social stimuli and most things that the normal person reacts to — ahh — they are seemingly more or less oblivious to.

THER.: Now let's go back — they react selectively to some social stimuli. Does this imply psychotic or neurotic behavior? Tell me more about that.

MOSS: Well, it is a very hard term to pin down. Let me start back there again — ah —

THER.: Start where?

MOSS: Chronic brain syndrome. I was simply commenting on the fact that there are at least three things wrong with these people, I suppose, and there can be more. One thing is they don't test in terms of the normal — they don't test according to the normal —(sighs)—

THER.: What did you say before about their test behavior?

---

[5] It is apparent that I have only a hazy idea of the CBS at this moment. Apparently what I am attempting to define is the typical chronic, backward patient in state hospitals.

Moss: It was variable. They tend to get abnormally low scores and this can be inferred from the fact that they would get average or above scores on other scales, do you see? So that's the first clue. The second clue is, of course, that they would — aren't ordinarily responsive to the average social stimuli, they are variable.

THER.: Can you give me an example?

Moss: When a nurse comes through she stops and says something to them and for the most part they don't pay any attention to her, or if they do pay attention, they interact in such a way that there's something about it which strikes one as being abnormal. And finally the fact that they, in terms of neurological examinations and things like that — that — is again termed as abnormal. For example, the EEG's and things like this. Reflexes, and so on.

THER.: Now this is how you would define CBS? Or this is what is given in lieu of something better?

Moss: I think I would go back to the statement that it often is given in hospitals when they lack some other definitive diagnosis to make. For example, the person doesn't appear to be depressive or he doesn't appear to be schizophrenic, the affect that he shows and the way he relates — there is something bizarre about him. But not quite to the degree of a person that is labeled schizophrenic. And a —

THER.: What's the actual definition of a chronic brain syndrome?

Moss: What's the actual definition?

THER.: Yes, how would a medical dictionary define it?[6]

Moss: I don't really know. I've been trying to think back on my own experience about people who were diagnosed as chronic brain syndrome, and ah, I must confess that this is a category that I haven't had much to do with in the last ten to twelve years, but obviously it is some sort of a brain impairment, a physiological impairment, either of the brain or the metabolism which feeds the brain — and I suppose it would ordinarily be turned up in a neurological examination, but the psychologist, or whoever does the test-

[6] "Chronic Brain Disorders ... result from relatively permanent, more or less irreversible, diffuse impairment of cerebral tissue function ... some disturbance of memory, judgment, orientation, comprehension and affect persists permanently." *Diagnostic and Statistical Manual: Mental Disorders,* Washington: American Psychiatric Association, 1952, p. 18.

ing, and ordinarily it is the psychologist, should find this scatter that I referred to —

THER.: Scatter? On the tests?

MOSS: Yes. Either that or a — person who is either of an advanced age or he has been hospitalized for a long period of time — ah — he might test very low on all of them, the different tests you give him. I guess I was earlier — again I find it a difficult category to establish. We can take people who have suffered some neurological impairment, some brain damage — these are people who suffer from things that I have, a stroke, for example — ah — and of course, in taking the social history you'd look for things that would substantiate the clinical evidence that you have gotten on the person.

THER.: What types of things would those be? Examples of their behavior?

MOSS: Well, ordinarily there would be two types of things: the things that were found out by the neurologist or the psychiatrist —

THER.: In their social behavior? Didn't you say that you would look for things in their social behavior?

MOSS: Right — and this would be the psychiatrist or things which would verify this diagnosis by testing.

THER.: How would you define this term, phenomenalistic?[7]

MOSS: Phenomenalistic. (Pause)

THER.: Especially as it applies to psychology and a means of measurement.

MOSS: Of course, there's a school of phenomenologists —

THER.: Who are the people in it?

MOSS: Well, the only one I can think of at the moment is called — Maniford Boss.[8]

THER.: I haven't heard that name in this school.

MOSS: As far as I can recall — would someone like Rogers be labeled a phenomenologist?

THER.: I don't know.

---

[7] "Phenomenology: The systematic investigation of phenomena or conscious experiences, especially as they occur immediately in experience, without implications." H. C. Warren, *Dictionary of Psychology,* Cambridge: Houghton-Mifflin Co., 1934, p. 199.

[8] Actually Boss is an existentialist. Also, it is Medard Boss.

Moss: What does phenomenology mean? The reason I think I know Boss's name is that again I ran across it in some studies on dreams.

Ther.: Oh, is he contemporary? I've been thinking more of historical names. Probably the names aren't so important, but defining it might be interesting.

Moss: What is a phenomenologist? Actually and again it is an inference from the term, I think it must be a person who sticks close to what he observes in people and doesn't attempt for the most part to make inferences about the person. He doesn't hypothesize various things about him.

Ther.: As opposed to what type of school that might do something like that?

Moss: As opposed to a psychoanalyst who takes what a person does and begins to immediately infer what it means "unconsciously" about the person.

Ther.: I thought that was what a phenomenologist might do, using the impression that a person gives them almost at face value.

Moss: Right. But does he infer a different level — of what a person does or what he says? I think he just takes it more or less at face value rather than making the inference to an underlying or covert "unconscious."

Ther.: Would it be helpful to have a tape recording of what you are saying? The reason I say that is because you might listen to it, and I might say, "Were you having any problem?," and you might say, "Yes, I was having a problem, but now that I listen to it I don't see that anyone else could pick that up."

Moss: What would be your inference as to whether I was or was not having problems? How do I appear to you *phenomenologically?*

Ther.: I would probably say that you didn't need any more therapy. As hard as we try and now and then we may cross an area, the problem comes up as to how close you are to the level you would like to get back to. That's very very hard to answer. You're probably the only one that could answer. Sometimes I might notice, very rarely, some words that a person with a Ph.D. wouldn't use, but I can't think of such a word at this moment. I wonder if at one time you hadn't used another word, but it's accurate. On this basis I don't think that you should still be in therapy.[9]

MOSS: There's a world of difference between what people don't know who listen to you and the judgments that you yourself make. As I've told you before I have used the tape recorder enough that I would more or less say that I appear normal to other people. Most of the tension is inward — it is actually in attempting to select the words that I am going to use and this occasions me much more difficulty than it did sixteen months ago. Always I am trying to get it across to other people the difficulty that I have in getting another person to understand.

THER.: You do sound normal, you don't make slips, people aren't lying to you when they say you sound perfectly normal.

MOSS: This has been told me again, and again, and again, and I didn't believe them until I actually made the recordings.

THER.: In having the anxiety about speaking, I am sure it can be handled with relearning many things, being stimulated by as much information as you can, and by speaking as much as you can, especially about things that are giving you trouble, which is what you are doing.

MOSS: Now I have the impression as I talk to you that I am more or less stumbling in comparison to the way I talked two years ago. I used to be much more spontaneous — now I am choosing every word, I am carefully selecting. This may be part of the reason that I am so anxious. If you attended to everything that you said in every detail, I think this would get to be very anxiety-arousing, but this is what I am doing. I am sure there are many subtle differences in the way I talk now and the way I talked earlier but I think it is largely in the quantity of speech. My impression in talking with you now is that my speech is much more halting than it was before, that earlier I would be much more fluent.

[9] I was flabbergasted at her conclusion, after having just suffered through half an hour of exquisite anxiety. On reflection I can possibly see how she arrived at her decision, based partly on preceding sessions and partly on her frustration in trying to handle a very difficult case. It is also just possible that I "snowed" her into believing that I had given adequate definitions. However, I still clung to speech therapy until the end of the spring semester.

THER.: I'll try to find a tape recorder and record what we talk about and it will provide a good comparison.

Moss: I think, a better way to do this, is that I am recording our talk right now —

THER.: You're speaking about —

Moss: If you want to listen to it you're welcome to do so [as I reach for my briefcase]. I've done this the last three or four times.

THER.: YOU ARE?! Good Grief![10]

III. Discussion

SIMPSON: Although there were still other therapeutic procedures, the preceding examples are typical and will serve to illustrate what speech therapy was all about. The goals of therapy were to obtain appropriate stimulation for Dr. Moss and to decrease his fears of venturing into his professional activities, which he had to reexplore. His attitude was both justified and not justified. His language ability was certainly adequate when compared to that of a normal population and even adequate when compared to that of a group of psychologists. It probably was not up to his pre-traumatic level. His desire to achieve perfection contributed to his fear. His occasional deficiency amplified his fear out of proportion.

Perhaps an analogy will clarify this point. All normal speakers have some dysfluencies. If the speaker considers himself to be normal, then the dysfluency does not bother him. If, however, the speaker considers himself to be a stutterer, then the dysfluency is a demonstration of his failure. All normal speakers also experience occasional word-finding problems. This seldom causes any reaction. However, if the speaker has had a language disorder, then any and all word-finding problems are signs of this disorder, which can cause fear.

As was stated, therapy continued throughout the next academic year. The goal was to help Dr. Moss reach the point where he could assume the major responsibility for his therapy, in essence, to become

[10] I had no intention of revealing the fact that I was recording our sessions at the present time, but I was still irritated by her judgment that I didn't need additional speech therapy, and wanted to bring home the fact that I already had tapes of our recent sessions. The mechanism for the "secret" recordings is revealed in the next chapter.

his own clinician. At the end of the spring semester (1969) it was recommended that he be dismissed with the option of returning if he felt the need. He did not feel the need, but has returned to give lectures to graduate students studying aphasia through the two succeeding years.

Therapy from my point of view has been successful — using the very broad definition of therapy. In this broad definition the major responsibility must finally be assumed by the aphasic himself and, in this sense, therapy will always be an on-going process. The success is aptly demonstrated in part by his present social and professional activities, in part by his continued professional growth, and in part by his proposed book on his personal encounter with aphasia.

Moss: I went to the university speech clinic from February, 1968 through May, 1969 (excluding time out for the summer period), or somewhere in the neighborhood of forty sessions. I saw three student therapists who functioned under the general direction of Dr. Robert Simpson. The difficulties for the poor student speech therapists who were saddled with a client who was at least as bright, far better educated, much more experienced, and of higher status than themselves, made for definite problems. Normally when that's the case, at least the client is so severely impaired in language that a good therapist-client relationship is cultivated anyway, but in my case I was at least equal in many interactions that went on in therapy and obviously that gave the student therapists some trouble in knowing what they were to be doing.

On the one hand I am very thankful that they didn't attempt to turn me away like many professional people that I contacted, on the rationale that after all I was so much better off than the majority of stroke patients. But on the other hand, even though they were receptive to my perception that I was going to pot in my occupation and to the potentiality for developing deeper-seated troubles, I still think that they were corrupted by having treated so many people with such severe disorders that they really didn't know how to "move upstream" and deal with the problems that I was having. In other words, they were skilled in teaching aphasics single words and getting them to read third-grade primers and teaching the rudiments of spelling, and so forth, but that wasn't the reason that I came to them.

What concerned me was the higher-order difficulties, so the approach with me was having me work at a much more complex level. They recognized that this was the case and they did their very best, but at times it left something to be desired. Thinking back about the experience, it would have benefited me if I had been coached to take the Graduate Record Exam, for example, where I would be under time pressure dealing with high-level vocabulary, analogies, and reading comprehension or some other equivalent type of test. The basic problem to me seems to be in integrating and organizing abstract-level verbal material rather than playing rote memory games. Finding a specific synonym for a word is terribly difficult, for instance; dealing instead with verbal analogies would lead me to just one word (e.g., A is to B as C is to X). I wouldn't be just sitting and grinding my wheels. If instead they had a whole series of reading-comprehension items that I could have worked through over time — trying to dig out the material or answering questions. In brief, it might have made more sense to tutor me as if I were going to take the GRE or the Miller's Analogy Test.

While they attempted to restructure the treatment session, making it much less of a patient-therapist relationship, they weren't always successful. I was too much an equal to the student therapists. This might have saved some defensive reactions on the part of the therapist as well as myself. Such statements are difficult for me in that I feel very kindly toward the speech department and their willingness to try to do something for such an atypical client as myself. I will always be grateful for the time and efforts of the three young women who listened so patiently to me and their responses in attempting to aid me. I especially appreciate the warm support Bob Simpson has always provided me. From my point of view, we all floundered at times, trying out various methods and techniques with a person who had already improved beyond the limits of most aphasics, but one who could not yet comfortably resume the role of an active professor. I frankly did not realize the amount of structure that went into my therapy until I read Dr. Simpson's report. He was quite correct in stating that part of my problem was bound up with the altered organization of the depleted brain neurons, and part of it was my reaction to the perceived consequences of my disabilities.

5

Two Years Later

By November of 1969 I could sum up my progress in the following way.

Underlying my difficulties in speaking, it seems to be that my filing system for the selection of words has become slightly out of kilter. Objectively, I speak normally now, except for occasionally floundering on a word or two. It is, most times, a slight semantic or meaning distortion. I haven't lost any language, I still have all the words that I ever had, but I no longer have the ability to recapture them as quickly as before. At such times I have to rely on the input of other people in conversation to lead me to them. Subjectively, I never had the impression that I had to reeducate myself in the language. There was never the sense of the speech therapist teaching me new (or forgotten) words. Therapy only stimulates the aphasic to produce the words that he still knows at some level. Psychologically this seems to be a matter of concentration; it takes far longer for me to develop an idea fully, and I still have difficulty in carrying a conception through to its completion.

If you are looking for difficulties in word-finding, as Bob Simpson put it, then you are bound to find them — even in normal people. I have also become very much aware that my frantic searching for words is not always reflected in my external appearance. People are often quite surprised if I confess to them the difficulty that I am experiencing in word-finding. Talking is something that the average indi-

vidual takes for granted (unless he is confronted with having to give
a formal speech), and I seldom gave it a second thought before my
accident.

During the past year the technique which probably has served me
best is a concealed tape recorder housed in an attaché case which can
be triggered by closing one of the clasps. My wife got it for me at
Christmas, 1968, at my request, and I secretly collected a large number of tapes of various interactions which I participated in, ranging
from highly informal contacts to classroom lectures and even speech
therapy. This led to an astonishing discovery for me: where I thought
my speech was poorly formed and suffering from chaotic lapses as I
frantically searched for words, I discovered that except for occasional
pauses, it sounded perfectly normal. I was amazed!

Bette states: "What he wanted was a little tape recorder that he
could put in his pocket — a little tiny thing like a pack of cigarettes,
and he could have the microphone on his tie clasp or pen. That was
fine for Dick Tracy or Mickey Spillane, but when you get down to
trying to find them, you can't, or if they do make them the microphone
isn't very sensitive. But finally I went to a hi-fi place and discovered
that you could take a small tape recorder (cassette) and put it in a
special attaché case which had a microphone in the handle. This was
great because Scott could carry the case with him, and whenever he
wanted to record, he only had to touch the handle and it would immediately start to record inside. It was sensitive and would pick up for
some distance. It has been a marvelous instrument for him because he
has been able to get conversations down without making notes. More
than that, I have attempted to point out to him time and time again
that in listening to his conversations you cannot tell who the aphasic is.
If you stop and listen to some other person, there are pauses and hesi-
tations while that person is gathering his thoughts. Nobody speaks as
though he is reading off a sheet of paper, but this is what Scott wants
to do and this is the way he used to do. He used to prepare lectures
ahead of time, study them, then simply make notes and follow his outline when he actually gave the talk. He gave marvelous addresses; people were always commenting on his ability to speak. But he took a lot
of time in his preparation. He has always done that, but it paid off.
Anyway, the recording of his conversations with other people should

really convince him that he doesn't block the way he thinks he does any more. Perhaps it is only his fear that he might block that causes him such anxiety. Of course, nobody can get inside his brain and know exactly how to change his own feelings. People whom we know now, who didn't know that he had had a stroke, are always amazed; they would never dream that anything like this had ever happened to him."

If I sounded normal, what then accounted for the tremendous rise in anxiety and the distorted perception during speaking? I have come to the conclusion that my reaction is actually related to my subjective effort to conjure up continually the words which I need to speak, and much of the tension is not evident to the other party. To help the reader empathize, it is as if an American were suddenly transported to a France where everyone speaks only French. Our hypothetical American had a couple of semesters of French in college, but now finds that all of his communications must be translated into the foreign language before he can make his needs, wishes, and thoughts known. In addition, he projects onto the situation the belief that he will suffer admonishment for each error he makes. (Everyone knows the attitude of many Frenchmen toward any foreigner who speaks their language less than perfectly.) The analogy begins to break down if you imagine that in thinking of concepts the American must first begin with the English equivalent; in my case, often I had no English words even to begin the translation, at least in the months following my stroke. Even now, two years later, the finding of words is at times most tenuous.

Despite this knowledge provided by the tapes, I am still prone to make misjudgments about my speaking ability — which shows that "insight" alone doesn't effect a cure. For example, Julie came to lunch the other day and asked if I could say "toy boat" three times. When I responded and became all mixed up in my pronunciation, the very first thing that came into my mind was a condemnation of my brain-addled tongue. Fortunately, I subsequently came to witness the fact that the other members of the family were similarly afflicted, but in a very real way this intropunitive obsession influences all of my dealings.

Anyone who has had a severe physical trauma — like the loss of a limb or eyesight or coordination — has a similar reaction, I'm sure, but I have no readily apparent disability, not even a partial paralysis, on which I can blame my incompetence. Despite Wepman's prediction that in time I would forget my stroke, the effects have always continued to plague me. Even the very fact that I feel compelled to write this autobiographical sketch reflects that I don't ever forget it for long.

Perhaps it would be well to spell out very concretely some of the types of memory difficulties that still concern me. I awaken each morning about 6:00 or 6:30 by my inner-alarm clock, get up, let out and feed the dog, and then listen to the 7 o'clock news on the "Today" show. It so happened that on a typical weekday morning recently I could not remember the master of ceremonies, even though the name seemed to be on the tip of my tongue. Finally, after worrying about it for twenty minutes or so, I turned to my wife, who had then awakened. She replied, "Think of UP" — at which I immediately provided "DOWNS." A few minutes later I was unable to come up with the name of the woman who cohosts the show with him. I again turned to my wife, who said (you can see by her responses that she is well used to this need to jog my memory): "What does a man do when he needs a HAIRCUT?" I at once answered, "He goes to see the hairdresser" (perseverating on the woman whose identity I sought). When I was told, "No, he sees the BARBER," I was then able to supply my wife with both the first and last names of Barbara Walters. These sorts of cues almost always sufficed since I was in a typical TOT (tip of the tongue) state. In quite a similar vein, I am always getting Johnny Carson of the "Tonight" show mixed up with the former star, Jack Paar. This happens to me now all the time in every field, not just in show business.

To continue a bit further with the "Today" show, here is an actual sample of my thought processes just as I attempted to write them down not long ago: "A couple of months ago they had on an olympic star, no, a decathalon winner. . . . Nope! She was an award-winning movie star. . . . What's it called? What is her name? . . . An Empy, huh uh! Emmy, yes, but that's an award for TV. . . . A gold statue (then a long pause, searching for the correct title, trying to picture an award-winning ceremony) . . . I'm really stumped . . . (then comes insight) AN OSCAR-WINNING STAR and her name is Patricia Neal. . . . But now I can't remember the book which she said will depict her struggle against brain damage." At this point I gave it up since the very real possibility existed that the name of the book never registered.

Or to make it more public, less subjective, bringing it much closer to home: for several weeks recently, I developed a habit of calling Mary Jo (my present secretary) by the name of Jo Ann (my former secretary), or of getting the names reversed and calling a colleague by his last name, "Paul," rather than his first name, "Gordie." (This is the price of having two first names, just as people upon first acquaintance tend to call me Moss for Scott or Dr. Scott or occasionally Dr. Moss Scott.)

When I used to complain about the ambiguousness of my memory, the response almost always elicited was, "Why, this happens to me all the time" (followed by a recitation of the last time that it happened). In time one gets turned off by this type of response. It is somewhat like a schizophrenic who tries to tell a behavior therapist about his delusions. The therapist ignores them and at some juncture the patient quits talking about them, in which case the symptom is rated cured. This habitual response to me indicates that most people try to deny the seriousness of what you are saying by relating it to something that occurs fairly frequently in the normal, everyday course of events. The loss of memory is familiar especially as we grow older, but it is a relative matter. It bothers me much, much more now that it did two years ago. The stroke suddenly aged me overnight both in memory and speaking. Reflectively, a conversation with me now reminds me of speaking with an elderly gentleman, say Bette's father — except that he often appears much more mentally agile than I. For someone who still cannot get his own children's names correct, the business of conducting professional affairs is a hazardous undertaking indeed.

In the spring of 1969 I entered into correspondence with the chief psychologist at a large V.A. hospital in the western part of the country about a possible position. I knew him casually and he was very responsive to my inquiry, in spite of the fact that he knew that I had suffered a stroke. I assured him of my almost complete recovery, which was in a sense the truth — I had recovered in excellent fashion, everything considered. In applying for any job I was faced with a peculiar dilemma. If I confronted a potential employer with what *I* perceived as my residuals, it might very well forestall any thoughts of hiring me (countless people had told me by this time that I grossly exaggerated my disabilities); on the other hand, I felt a failure to do so was a misrepresentation of myself with consequent guilt about the duplicity and the fact that I would soon be found out. I tried to stipulate that I was interested in a clinical-type position, one which I felt competent to handle, but when the offer came it was for a job as the chief program evaluator of the hospital, with the promise that in a short time I would be promoted to the vacant chief research psychologist's position.

Because of my abiding interests in research, I almost accepted that position in spite of the many doubts that it immediately raised; however, there were other factors that made me hesitate. I felt loyalty to the director of clinical psychology at Illinois and he was currently on a six-month sabbatical and would not return until fall. During his absence I held down several fairly responsible duties. Then my mother underwent another heart failure just at the time of the final decision. She was hospitalized for a month and her physician informed us that more than likely her illness would be terminal (fortunately it wasn't). But in the final analysis, my many doubts about myself persisted and I was simply unconvinced that I could accept such a responsible position. I eventually turned it down.

So in the fall of 1969 I again entered into my academic job, even though I had many reservations about continuing it. It soon became apparent that I could not promote the community mental health (community psychology) program in the way that I had been hired to do. Even though I was convinced of a strong public service orientation and believed that psychologists, among other professionals, should be responsible to meet the problems growing out of great social needs, it was impossible to make and sustain the numerous contacts which would be required in promoting an expanding community program. As the first semester neared its end, I forfeited the leadership to another staff member. In discussion of my future role with the director and the chairman of the department, it was decided that in the coming year, 1970-71, I would give up entirely attempting to teach community psychology and substitute instead two successive sections of abnormal psychology, while still keeping a laboratory on psychotherapy. It was some small consolation knowing that probably I could handle large didactic courses in abnormal much better than the less structured seminar courses with bright graduate students.

My primary reason for coming to the university was to teach clinical graduate students some of the things that I had learned over the past seventeen years, particularly what I had been doing in relation to community mental health in the previous six years. There was no way of knowing that even without a stroke much of what I knew (or thought I knew) would be discounted because in my orientation I was considered to be a representative of the "old school" in contrast to the new militant behaviorism (see Chapter 7).

However, a strong, secondary reason for my having chosen Illinois was that it would bring me once again into contact with Charlie Osgood and the possibility that we could collaborate on a book that I had in mind. We had had a half-dozen contacts in the first few weeks after I arrived, and had already come to the conclusion that the majority of writing must be left to me, since he was (as usual) tremendously overcommitted. After the accident and the resulting aphasia, the possibility of my doing any writing seemed remote. But eight months later, out of desperation and seeking yet another form of self-help, I began to dictate to my wife the beginning outline of the book.

The book gradually took on a structure and form somewhat different from what I had originally intended, since I was no longer capable of writing with nearly the style or spontaneity that I had two years earlier. However, when one gets to the point of writing a book, much of the material is already on hand in thought and on paper. The book as it was transformed became a casebook composed of a dozen previously handled cases selected from among those in my files, some of which had already been reported in various professional journals. All that was really left for me to do was to put the cases in some sort of logical order, and to write three chapters: an introduction and two other integrative chapters, one on the experimental and one on the clinical aspects of exploring dream symbolism with hypnosis. After all, this had been part of my clinical practice for twenty years and I should have been thoroughly familiar with it. On the other hand, absolutely nothing came to me as easily as it had two years before — neither the thoughts nor how to unify them nor how to translate them from my head into written language. But my wife and I plugged away, having plenty of time since my professional activities and our social activities were greatly curtailed.

At the appropriate time, Charlie sat down and prepared a critique of the book for me and then wrote a foreword to it. We decided that I should approach the University of Illinois Press, both because it had published Osgood's initial text on the semantic differential (*The Measurement of Meaning,* 1957), and because I had neither the energy nor the poise to enter into protracted negotiations with other publishers. As it turned out, the editors of the press were very receptive to the book, and accepted it for publication (*Dreams, Images, and Fantasy: A Semantic Differential Casebook,* 1970). They also wished to publish a supplemental paperback book prepared on the treatment of an illustrative phobic case (*Black Rover, Come Over*), written largely by the patient herself, along with an accompanying tape of selected episodes from the actual psychotherapeutic sessions.[1] In my judgment the two books were reasonably well written, but the content often had to be rather painfully dredged from my reduced intellectual and language capacity. Incidentally, I again played a little game with myself and the publishers and never mentioned my brain damage to them.

So two years after my stroke I am beginning to work as hard at my professional duties as I was earlier, but accomplishing less. Although I now do much of my work at home rather than in the office, I nevertheless am busy at my typewriter or listening to tapes or composing lectures four or five hours each day, including Saturday and Sunday. I am amused at my halfhearted attempts to "take it easy" in the face of the habits of a professional lifetime. Even though I still toy with the idea of retiring to a tropical beachside hut, I don't think I will ever make it. The demands for a full-time and active life are impossible to avoid within the constraints of a slight impairment. In recent months, I have become aware that my physical tempo has begun to pick up and at times bears a resemblance to the hectic manner in which I used to balance at least a half-dozen tasks at once. This increased activity still feels strange and rather uncomfortable and as soon as I am aware of what I am doing I attempt to slow down, but little by little I seem to be getting back into the old acrobatic mold.

Quite by chance, it was pointed out to me by one of my students

---

[1] The *Black Rover* tape, by the way, is a reasonably good sample of my premorbid personality and the accompanying patterns of thought and speech.

that I had "unconsciously" learned to compensate partially for my handwriting disability. By this time I had learned to sign my name without embarrassing halts and jerks and without the last letters disintegrating into inconspicuous marks. But what was pointed out to me when I was signing a curriculum card was that the index finger of my left hand seemingly steadied (actually it pushed against) the right hand which held the pen. I was amazed when this was pointed out; I had no realization that I was doing this to compensate for the loss of power and mobility in the afflicted hand. Later I noticed that I did this habitually. However, at the time it happened, I took some hidden pride in the fact that I immediately came forth with the rationalization that this was the way I had learned in early childhood to write across a page without lines, and then we laughed at the odd ways children learn to write. In the time ahead, with a little practice, I learned to sign my name without the extra effort supplied by the member of the opposite hand, thus doing away with another sign that might give me away. This works fine as long as I don't have to sign my name several times in a row. If it is required that a sentence or two be written, I almost always, on some pretext, give the pencil and pad to another person.

Having been sensitized to the automatic way that my body compensated for my right hand, I then looked at other related features, and discovered that in my gardening I now made adjustments so that the left hand would take on most of the more intricate or demanding tasks, and in driving the car I now tended to steer with the left hand. The right hand was still functional in most activities but quite involuntarily the other hand had begun to replace it in the more arduous or complicated jobs.

In some ways I was extremely fortunate that the stroke occurred in the university setting, since the faculty had been so tolerant of my limitations during my recovery. On the other hand, I was suddenly very impressed with the limited financial resources that are available to a severely handicapped person in this society. I had slowly built up a private life insurance program which would modestly protect my wife and family in the event of my death, but it never occurred to me that I should take out some form of wage insurance as well, since I had never been hospitalized in my life except for a short episode in the service.

I had given up my disability retirement based on more than sixteen years of federal employment and my federal health insurance when I came to Illinois. I had the foresight to take out a fairly expensive family health insurance which covered about 80 percent of my hospital bills (which came to almost $1,000 for less than two weeks' hospitalization). Inadvertently, I had skipped the group insurance policy, but thought that I would pick it up at the next eligibility period; however, when I tried to obtain coverage after my accident, I was politely but firmly turned down.

In terms of the university's retirement system, during the first five years of employment, rather than receiving a disability annuity, employees are provided with a lump-sum cash benefit equal to half the salary received during the term of employment. For me this meant that if I were declared disabled after two full years I could receive approximately $20,000 paid over two following years. In the back of my mind was the concern that I really was worth much more dead than permanently disabled. My Social Security was paid up (44 quarters) but there was the qualification there that in cases of disability you had to be covered in five of the last ten years. I was covered for 1959-60-61 before I returned to federal service, so I had to sweat out paying two additional years from the small income that I derived from my two earlier books, which I did in the early springs of 1969 and 1970. This made me eligible for a small stipend in case of permanent and total disability. This is why I wanted to return to federal service and to complete at least my twenty years, which would qualify me for a part-time pension if I had another accident. Security for my family was my overwhelming objective.

My experience brought home to me the wisdom of having a federally sponsored national health and disability insurance program which everyone would be required to join. After all, I am a living example of the fact that absolutely no one can tell that he might not, today or tomorrow, suffer from an accident that would partially or totally disable him, with a catastrophic result in most cases, both for the individual and most or all of the people who are dependent upon him. On the other side of the coin, insecurity can be a prime motivating factor. One never knows how much he can do until he is forced by circumstances to do it.

6

Formative Influences

There have been relatively few people who have written accounts of their aphasia, and among the handful that have, no one, to my knowledge, has gone into the factors of his own growth and development as background to his eventual cerebral trauma (see Chapter 10). One can view a stroke, heart attack, or cancer as simply very unfortunate accidents that happen to befall some people; on the other hand, it seems reasonable to me that perhaps certain personalities may develop certain types of disorders. My professional career over twenty years had evolved in a fairly promising way — was the stroke the eventual consequence of this very high level of activity? And why me rather than a hundred aspiring other colleagues?

Are there more personal ties between the formative influences in childhood and adolescence and the ultimate brain damage? Or was it just an accident, such as befalls a person walking down the street who is hit by a speeding car, or did some aspect of my history pre-dispose me eventually to develop a vascular disease process? Was it due to the rich diet brought on by being a member of this affluent society (I have always been partial to chocolate, ice cream, and other sweets)? Was it due to stress or diet or constitutional or heredity factors or did it simply just happen? I may be looking too hard for an answer when no objective information exists at the present time. Since I don't have the perspective nor the facts to answer the question, I must leave it for later, better educated, and more sophisticated persons.

I

I was born May 17, 1924, the only child of parents of European extraction. My mother was twenty-five and my father forty-six. My birth was a hazardous affair, since the diminutive size of my mother (4′ 8″, 98 pounds) made delivery difficult, and forceps had to be used. I still retain a perceptible frontal head indentation from this experience. No serious aftereffects were apparent, however, as my general health during infancy and childhood was good. My disposition is reported to have been remarkably cheery — I was a happy, smiling baby who seldom fussed or cried, at least according to my mother's account. I began teething at four months and took my first unaided steps at ten months. However, I did not speak with any facility until around two and a half years, at which time my mother says that I started out with more or less complete sentences. I contracted the usual childhood diseases, chicken pox, mumps, and measles, in that order. I never incurred any broken bones. Hence, there appears to have been no special susceptibility to accident or illness, aside from a tendency to catch the common cold. I averaged two or three long sieges each winter, interspersed with severe sore throats all during my childhood and early youth.

The only accident of consequence ever to befall me in childhood happened when I was six, at which time I tripped while playing and hit my forehead on a brick. A contusion or concussion resulted, rendering me unconscious for about 30 hours. I was told that I vomited every half hour and that that saved me from an operation — a belief which is, of course, an example of "folk medicine." When I came out of it I can vaguely remember that my mother told me she was going downtown, and asked whether there was anything that she could bring me. I answered no, because I was still too ill, but by the time she returned I had already recovered enough to react with disappointment that she had not brought me a toy cowboy pistol with silver bullets. I was never hospitalized until military service, when I entered the hospital for treatment of a mastoid infection, for a tonsillectomy (which got rid of my sore throats), and because of measles.

The socioeconomic status of my family can be categorized as lower to middle class. We moved frequently during my formative years and the number of dwellings occupied totaled seventeen: rooms, apartments, and houses. I was born in Newark, New Jersey, and for several months, I am told, we resided in a three-room apartment. Our financial standing at this time was at its highest peak — my father's income averaged from $150 to $200 a week, which was a considerable sum in those days. When we were physically able, my mother and I went back to her home town of Baraboo in southern Wisconsin, while my father resumed his tour of the country as a newspaper columnist. In Baraboo we were joined by my mother's mother, a widow who, since her husband's death many years before, had relied upon her four children for support. Our first house there had nine rooms, our second, ten. In both places my mother rented out some of the rooms.

When I was three, Mother decided to move to Madison, a change necessitated by the sporadic financial support provided by my father. There my mother, grandmother, and I settled into a six-room flat in the university district and took student roomers. Mother also enrolled in business and secretarial courses at the city vocational school, hoping to obtain a high school diploma and eventually some sort of an office position. Three years later, at the behest of my father, we moved into a higher-class neighborhood and gave up taking roomers. Father insisted that our former residence cast reflections on him and the family name and that if we would move, financial support would be forthcoming. A year later, when the promised support failed to materialize, we were forced to move back into a less expensive house. This time it was a four-room flat near mother's new job as a bookkeeper and cashier in a downtown restaurant. In 1934 we moved to yet another four-room apartment a few blocks away; it was then that my parents were divorced. I was ten years old at this time and in fifth grade, and I felt ashamed and kept the secret of the divorce from my friends as long as I could.

In the spring of 1936 my mother married a chef at the restaurant where she was employed. He soon persuaded her that the West

Coast provided excellent opportunities for employment, so within three months we headed west, while grandmother rented a room and remained in Madison. Unfortunately, we arrived in California at a time when a great westward migration was developing and employment was scarce. My stepfather managed to find work in the famous Brown Derby, but my mother was unable to find a job. The troubled economic situation combined with personal conflicts between my stepfather and me resulted in increasing dissension, and within six months my mother and I fled back to Madison.

Mother rented a room for us and soon succeeded in finding employment. Two weeks later a reconciliation was effected between my mother and stepfather, who followed her back to the Midwest. We moved into a larger apartment, but four months later my step-father, again dissatisfied, persuaded my mother to move to Chicago. Since it was summer vacation time, I spent most of my time with my grandmother or visiting relatives in Iowa. In the fall my stepfather decided that Dayton, Ohio, would be an attractive city in which to try his luck, so once again we were on the move. Both parents this time succeeded in getting jobs and we settled down in a two-room apartment to spend the winter.

Following the advent of the new year, however, we returned to Madison once more — largely at the insistence of my mother, who was none too fond of Dayton. Upon our return we moved into a two-room and then a three-room apartment. It was then that my parents decided to purchase, on time, a big, antiquated, student rooming house, which remained in the family until seven years ago. This house had twenty rooms, and because of its age it was constantly in need of repair and renovation. But my stepfather couldn't contain his wanderlust, and within a year he set off again to search for more profitable employment. This time, however, mother stayed behind to operate their newly acquired establishment. The year following, she instigated divorce proceedings against her absentee husband — the divorce being granted when I entered the eleventh grade.

II

So the household in which I grew up consisted of my mother, my grandmother, and occasionally my father or stepfather, and a constant assortment of roomers. My father was a small and exceedingly thin individual, with a high-strung, immature, and self-indulgent personality. He was a supersalesman whose chief business was selling himself and his newspaper column to editors throughout the country. But whatever his talents as a writer, he had none as a husband and a father. He simply did not know the meaning of responsibility, faithfulness, or honesty. He used up every penny of his income, and more, on women and at the race tracks (he was a compulsive gambler, arranging his business to follow the tracks, going south in the winter and north in the summer).

One of his few redeeming features was his abhorrence of alcohol, or so I considered it until I came eventually to recognize that it was due to his addiction to narcotics. (Mother referred obliquely to his addiction, and later I discovered a hypodermic syringe among his things, although I do not know what substance he used.) He smoked three packs of Bull Durhams and drank two dozen cups of black coffee a day. Despite the fact that his eating habits were miserable, his health was amazingly good. He seldom knew a sick day until, at the age of fifty-nine, he had a heart attack. He was divorced from mother by this time, and he continued to make a living of sorts as a "broker" (bookmaker) on the West Coast, until he died in 1953, just before my graduation from Illinois. He had sent as a present a slightly used marble ashtray with a horse in the middle. The horse was broken, and while he had, typically, insured the item for $50, the Post Office evaluated it at $12.50.

My relationship with my father was obviously never close. I seldom saw him for more than a week or two a year before the divorce, and thereafter only four times more. He was twenty years older than my mother, and on the infrequent occasions when we got together he attempted comradely gestures, but our interests as well as our ages were too far apart. His idea of a good time was to take me on a tour of the big cities which he knew so well. To me he appeared more like a benevolent once-or-twice-a-year Santa Claus than a real flesh-and-blood father. But as a young boy I remember wanting to feel proud of him. I built him up in the eyes of my boyhood acquaintances, portraying him as a famous syndicated newspaper columnist.

A particularly revealing insight occurred during our last meeting in the summer of 1948. After not having seen me for over nine years, he spent most of our time alone delivering a highly belated lecture on sex, women, and marriage. He concluded by saying, "Women are delightful little creatures, God bless them, you couldn't get along without them; but you've got to feed them a line all the time, build them up, make them think they're important. Yes, sir, sex, I mean marriage, is the most wonderful thing in the world." Incidentally, I was a "junior," and I took to calling myself by my middle name, Scott, shortly after his death.

In many ways my mother was the antithesis of my father. A product of a small-town, middle-class, German upbringing, she was essentially a warm and responsible individual, not the least of her virtues being a tremendous capacity for work, despite a rheumatic heart condition which had plagued her since childhood. In addition to duties ordinarily entailed in the maintenance of a household and in raising a son, she also took in roomers and at the same time held down a full-time office job. But such is not the full measure of her devotion and industriousness. For eleven years she also had the sole responsibility of caring for and nursing her sick mother.

Mother spent as much time with me as her numerous activities would allow, and my character is largely the result of her interest in my welfare. During her free time she read, told stories, or just played games with me. When I went to grade school, she was an active member of the P.T.A.; her efforts were unceasing in trying to give me anything I desired that she could afford. When I was in high school, she was never too tired to press my clothes, bake a cake, or make sandwiches for some group of friends I might bring home. Despite the hard work, she had retained much of the petite attractiveness which had acquired for her a modeling job with Singer Sewing Machines when she was younger.

While I felt love, responsibility, and respect toward her, I seldom confided in her or came to her for advice. Ours was never a confidential relationship. Perhaps it was because our relationship was never really intimate that we got along so well together. Her father was murdered when she was eleven, and as she remembers it, she had been the "apple of his eye." In later years I became aware that in some ways, I reminded her of him. I think that she sought to lavish on me all the warmth and attention of a mother, a frustrated wife, and a little girl whose need for a loving father was thwarted. But this is all inferential.

My mother's second husband, the cook at the restaurant where she was employed, was a downstate Indiana farmboy and in many ways the direct opposite of my idealized fiction father. He had little of the suave worldliness which characterized my father — he was as much a "physical" specimen as my father was a "personality" type. Our relationship was always cool and restrained. He made only feeble attempts to gain my friendship and confidence, and for the most part we avoided contact. For mother's sake, I made what I considered to be concessions in the direction of a peaceful relationship with him, but as I think back he doubtlessly considered my actions as those of a spoiled little brat, which probably they were. The jealousy which our rivalry for my mother's affections engendered probably contributed subsequently to their separation and divorce five years later.

Mother died of congestive heart failure a few months after our move back to California. She was until the end a devotee of an admixture of Presbyterianism, Unity, and spiritualism. I recall a funny little story from before I was caught up in professional ethics. When I came back from military service she tried to persuade me to see one or another of her spiritual advisors. Finally, one Saturday night, my date and I agreed to see a medium. This woman, as I remember it, wore a large turban to help conceal the fact that she was bald. We were ushered in separately and she spoke in typically ambiguous terms to me, probably in the hope that I would project and amplify onto them, which, of course, I wasn't about to do. Eventually she recognized my skepticism and said she couldn't focus on the supernatural because of my lack of belief. We ended the session on a note of mutual distrust.

My date went in next, while I sat alone in the anteroom. Shortly thereafter I was joined by a weary young woman who, it turned out, was the medium's daughter, who had just finished work at a local laundry. She complained of a headache. Having recently learned something of hypnosis at the university, I volunteered the information that I knew something of the technique of relieving tension headaches, if only she would attend for a few minutes to what I had to say. She proceeded to enter hypnosis, which I labeled as 'progressive relaxation" without mentioning the term "hypnotism," whereupon I quizzed her extensively about her mother. At the conclusion she promptly forgot about the conversation upon my suggestion of amnesia, and awoke without the headache. When my date came out, I mentioned to the medium that I, too, often had intuitions about people, and proceeded to reveal in my best Svengali-like manner part of what I had learned. We ended up in quite an animated discussion which lasted an additional hour; out of it I received an invitation to address the advocates of the spiritual church (which I declined) and an offer to excuse my contribution for her services (which I accepted).

I never did tell my mother of the specific interactions that had ensued, but it always struck me as strange that she continued firm in her belief in spiritualism, especially since through my training as a psychologist I had other interpretations which I would have been happy to share; but there was nothing I could do or wanted to do to dissuade her from her beliefs. Each of us has many different systems for making life (and death) more acceptable.

Basically, I think my skepticism sprang from the fact that at the age of eight or nine I became interested in magic, sorcery, and slight-of-hand, and all through high school I was an enthusiastic, though quite amateur, practicing magician. Having savored the art of producing baffling effects or illusions through seemingly inexplicable powers, I in turn came to have an extremely doubting attitude toward others who attributed their exploits to the supernatural. In the last analysis, I reasoned that everything must have a rational (scientific) explanation, even though it may not be apparent at the moment. This was my faith. I also think that this was the reason why, in my present crisis, I fell back on intellectualizations as a bulwark rather than reverting to my earlier childhood belief in God.

The last individual to figure prominently in our household relationships was my grandmother. Aside from the relatively short period when my mother was married to my stepfather, grandmother was almost always a member of the immediate family. I remember her initially as a kind old lady, whose authority was not to be taken too seriously. Her social life centered about the sewing circle of the Christ Presbyterian Church. Following a stroke at age seventy-two which paralyzed the left side of her body (she was left-handed), she came to live with us, and remained until she died almost twelve years later. (She was not affected by aphasia, which demonstrates once more that in left-handed people the speech center is often located in the left hemisphere.) Despite her affliction, she managed to retain a large amount of good nature and aside from infrequent periods of dejection, she maintained a seemingly high level of morale during the first few years. Mentally and physically she remained active. She was up and about every day, puttering about the house, setting the table, washing dishes, and even preparing a meal or baking a pie.

Through the years, however, she became increasingly enfeebled as she suffered more strokes, and the task of taking care of her and nursing her during her increasingly frequent spells of choking became greater — it became a longtime, grueling, and grim job. I used to imagine that she deliberately snoozed during the day so that she could keep my mother awake during the long nights. Grandmother gradually developed a typical invalid psychology with its accompanying expressions of dependency and unceasing demands.

Not until early adulthood did I fully realize the parasitic relationship that my grandmother had always exercised upon my mother. As I gradually weaned the story from my mother, it was totally disillusioning. Since the time my mother was old enough to work at age fifteen, she had always been burdened with responsibility for grandmother. Grandmother actually had a very domineering personality. Mother claimed much later that grandmother had arranged for her to marry my father because he was well-to-do and gave grandmother sums of money. Both my grandmother and my father were the same age; theoretically they might have married each other.

As a result I became increasingly bitter toward my grandmother and my attitude toward her changed from ambivalence to downright rejection. Symptomatic of these largely suppressed feelings is the fact that from tenth grade until I went into the service I literally had to force myself to eat at the table with my grandmother. I much preferred to eat alone in the living room under the pretext of listening to the evening news. Her clicking dentures filled me with nausea. This was the closest and only contact with a stroke victim in my young life;

who knows what lasting hostile feelings were built up by this early learning? How much of my intropunitiveness do I now take out on myself?

III

My interest in sexual matters began when I was six and my curiosity impelled me to discover the anatomical differences between myself and a little neighbor girl, which in turn led to my first trauma — the girl confessed to her mother. The second instance happened the same year, when my mother caught me in the new-found experiment of masturbating. But these two experiences did not pave the way for any eventual sexual conflicts, although they were probably instrumental in arriving at the decision that I couldn't talk about sex or other important personal items with my mother. I liked girls from a very early age and I matured quite young — I began shaving when I was twelve.

I think I was too socialized even at an early age to engage in blatantly asocial acts, though this didn't inhibit my enjoyment of the antics of other selected friends. It is true that for a short time when I was nine or ten I was a member of a "sex club," the main activity of which was the collection of dirty pictures, until someone stole our scrapbook; and I slipped into my share of movies about that time (the price was only a dime but the adventure was the thing, and we did engage in some ingenious schemes). I even engaged in some petty shoplifting, until I got caught. In high school I took up with a collection of friends who periodically assembled in the basement of a "boy chemist," where we sat around inhaling nitrous oxide (laughing gas) or manufacturing a mixture which, when dried, made an explosive that we went about sprinkling beneath the tires of parked cars or putting in measured amounts in safety zones. Occasionally I used to help steal a few needed chemicals from the University of Wisconsin laboratories.

Brutus and his special acquaintance, Red, were the closest I came to being embroiled in pure delinquency. One summer evening I was in Brutus's third-floor apartment when he happened to see a young woman in an adjacent apartment building lounging about in her pajamas. He turned off the light and when she flopped on her stomach on her bed to read a book, he pried the screen off his window and proceeded to shoot the lady in the buttocks with his B-B gun. She came to the window and Brutus was drawing another bead when I mischievously turned on the light. She called the police. When they arrived, we went down the back stairs, got on our bikes, and rode furiously into a jammed intersection with the police in close pursuit. We eventually escaped by riding full throttle into the open door of an ice cream parlor, where the manager, with whom we had established a close financial relationship, hid us out (we usually went there to partake of ice cream delicacies after our paper routes). The police, of course, had Brutus's address, but to his credit he didn't squeal on me.

Both Brutus and Red were also involved with explosives, but to a more serious degree. I can remember the time one early morning when they rousted me out of bed and took me down to one of the lakes and "as the sun rose over the water" blew the end off one of a university sorority's piers. This was their Fourth of July celebration! Or the time we went walking around Madison's Capital Square and they chucked a lighted dynamite cap under the homemade tent of an elderly gentleman who used to charge a nickel for writing your name in an old-fashioned artistic scroll. Brutus went through a period when he was addicted to finding out everything he could about ballistics. He eventually turned from library studies to building miniature artillery. The announced intention was to blow the dome off the state capitol. I was invited along with Red one day when they tried out a newly constructed cannon. It partially backfired and brought down a stucco wall against which it was anchored; the projectile which they had loaded in the front blew out the window of a ladies' tea room. Both Brutus and Red were arrested and eventually placed on probation, while I faded quietly into the crowd.

Eventually Brutus was placed on second probation when he was caught after a series of midnight chases dressed as a batman who went about scaring college lovers in the university woods. He eventually went into the merchant marines, and after the war faked a college diploma and obtained a job on the faculty of an enginering school. So far as I know he is still succeeding. Red didn't turn out nearly so well. He got mixed up in a very unhappy marriage. He commandeered a taxi to take him to another state (this was before the days of the pirating of commercial airliners) and ended up in the cab as a potential suicide with a .38 automatic. He was shipped off to the nearby mental hospital and I lost track of him after that. I feel fortunate in that if these events had happened in this age, I would probably have been hauled off to some court and been labeled a juvenile delinquent. This could have been a choice point in life which might have prevented me from eventually going into psychology.

A wonderful "first love" preoccupied me for over five years, from the beginning of tenth grade through two years of Army service. I was obsessed with a girl several years my junior. She lived on my paper route, and I took every opportunity to be with her, dreamed about her at night, and fantasized about her during the daytime. And most important, our relationship had little or nothing to do with sex in its purely physical manifestation.

Our relationship, once it became known, evoked censure from both of our parents and much comment from the neighbors, who saw us constantly together. Our meetings became progressively more clandestine; and we met secretly up the block or in the evening. As a consequence we shared little of our "social life" with others — a life which consisted of long walks, bike riding, and very infrequent movies. I was willing to give up my friends to be with her. The relationship filled many important and satisfying roles for me. Her father had been an alcoholic who had committed suicide when she was eleven; I therefore saw myself as attempting partially to fill his shoes; she had an older brother who used to be quite mean to her on occasion, and I tried to protect her from his wrath. But most of all, I was her sweetheart and she was a delightful, lovely young girl who was budding into early maturity. The love and affection that I felt for her was the most altruistic one that I was capable of giving.

When I eventually lost her at nineteen, I was, needless to say, very distraught. I mourned the loss of a relationship which had played such a frankly momentous part in my life. But there were many obstacles to our eventual happiness: while she did grow into a beautiful young lady, she was somewhat sickly; the number of interests we could have shared would have been limited; she was a staunch Catholic; and so on. At least these were the rationalizations that I used to combat my depression.

IV

I attended nine educational institutions between first grade and college. The overall effect of such rapid changes in school resulted in an imperfect grounding in many basic subjects, which was compensated to some extent by my ability to make varied social relationships. My schooling was marked by my limited performance in contrast to my potential ability. My memory actually began to function in an organized fashion about the fifth year. I can remember the intelligence test I had to take before I was admitted to kindergarten. The test consisted of following a woman from room to room, watching her actions and then going back and repeating them in detail. Happily I passed and started to school. In second grade, I was a very poor reader and had to attend a special reading class after school. I was quite ashamed of this and always came late to class so that the other children would not see me going into the school room. I also re- member, vaguely, that I had something like a facial tic during those first few years.

In the summer between third and fourth grade we had moved to another school, and it was during this period I first realized the import of human mortality. I spent some of my time during the hot summer days lying in the shade of our cool back porch. One afternoon my boyish mind turned to the problem of God and the hereafter. It was then I first realized that some day my mother and I must both die. It frightened me terribly, this insight into the frailty of flesh. I cried for an hour or more, but my thoughts were well hidden and I never told anyone.

The next year we moved to still another school and I entered fifth grade. I was simply too immature, and at the end of the first term the teacher demoted me back to 4B for a "lack of seriousness in approach to my studies." A general achievement test administered at this time indicated that I possessed sufficient knowledge to do ad- vanced work. Mother cried and said it was her fault for starting me so young, and I can remember trying to console her and resolving to do better. I was shamefaced about going back to school and having to sit among the fourth graders. During grade school, several teachers remarked that I was apparently inclined to become hyperactive.

In junior high I continued as a mediocre student, but had no special difficulty until ninth grade, when I encountered algebra. A pronounced computational disability then became apparent. I passed both algebra and geometry with D— grades, largely because I had as a private tutor a friend of the teacher's, and after geometry I faithfully promised the teacher I would never take another math course again. In tenth grade I received my only outright failure. This was brought about by an unfortunate personality conflict with the teacher in combination with a subject vastly uninteresting to me, the essentials of English grammar. I made up the grade in summer school by studying Shakespearian plays.

Perhaps the greatest significance was my progressive raise in grades, from a C average in ninth grade to an A— average in twelfth grade. This improvement was due to the fact that until tenth grade my primary motivation was in athletics; for example, in ninth grade I won seventeen points in the city track and field meet. But in the tenth grade I was declared ineligible for sports because of my poor grades. I had matured early, and while this gave me temporary physical superiority, I stopped growing when I was twelve. Also, for the first time in my life we had a permanent home, and I actually went for more than two semesters to the same school. I graduated forty-first out of a class of 191 students and won a small award for being the most improved student over a three-year period. In this connection it is of interest to note the progressive rise in my intelligence quotient. It was measured as an IQ of 114 in kindergarten; 126 on the Terman scale in eighth grade; and a Wechsler IQ score of 137 in twelfth grade. I also had some special aptitude in art and dramatics.

I went into military service in December, 1942, and I would characterize my three and a half years in the Air Corps as sometimes instructive, often interesting, and, all things considered, a tremendous waste of time. I transferred to sixteen different bases, went through basic training three times, attended six schools, including the Army Specialized Training Program for a while in chemical engineering (where I successively failed college algebra, trigonometry, and calculus), and ended up doing largely trivial and routine Air Force ordnance work. I was on Guam when the war ended. When discharged, I enrolled at the University of Wisconsin, majoring in psychology in March, 1946.

By carrying a heavy schedule, I managed to do four years of work in two and a half years, graduating with a B.S. degree in August, 1948. I then transferred to the University of Illinois, where I obtained my Ph.D. five years later. My grades averaged 4.7 points (out of a possible 5 points) in college. For a long period of time I answered inquiries as to why I had chosen to go into clinical psychology as attributable to the fact that the ship which brought me home from the Pacific was named the *Dorothea L. Dix* (after a lay person who had much to do with the founding of state hospitals in this country before the turn of the century), which was the most fanciful explanation that I could arrive at.

I guess I went into clinical psychology because I had a strong motivation to help myself and others. In 1948 I wrote, "I find very little attraction to academic psychology and research per se, and am almost wholly interested in psychology from the viewpoint of a practicing clinician." The Strong Vocational Interest Test revealed that at the time my highest ratings were for jobs similar to those of a personnel manager, a YMCA secretary, and a minister. A low secondary field of interest was in psychology. I would be remiss not to mention the influence which one person had on me, an experimental psychologist interested in communications theory, Charles Osgood. I ended up doing my dissertation, "The quantitative semantic analysis of dreams in psychotherapy," under Charlie. I never worked so hard for a year and a half as I did for him, but out of this came a newly won respect for research (and statistical methods) and it changed the future course of my professional life. He personified perfection and he demanded this quality from his subordinates. From then on I was a clinical (later a community) psychologist with a strong personal interest in applied research.

V

Because of our frequent moves and since I did not have a father or even a mother whom I felt I could confide in, I was thrust back increasingly upon reliance on my own inner self. I learned to adjust to a variety of transitory social relationships but to adopt long-standing friendships cautiously. I was essentially a loner in many of my accomplishments. To the world I learned to effect a mask of cheerfulness, calmness, and tolerance; inside I was often bewildered, but somehow had come to believe that I shouldn't evidence this disquietude to other people. While I seldom developed real feelings of trust and confidence in other men, I did manage to develop a series of intensive and extended relationships with women. I almost always had a girl with whom I could exchange confidences and who, consequently, knew me better than most people. Even in those cases I seldom discussed in detail my feelings of self-doubt and inferiority. I may be grossly oversimplifying, but in growing up I was clearly concerned about my lack of height (I was 5′ 6″ tall), and much of my activity was in direct compensation, first in athletics and later in scholarship. For whatever reason, I was determined not to be just another nameless member of society — I had to be someone special. As a result, I persevered far longer in staying with an assigned task than most other people. At the same time it was always characteristic of me to blame myself rather than others for any failures or shortcomings. Yet somehow, through the years, I seemed to grow measurably in emotional maturity.

In 1953 I took my first job after graduation, at a V.A. hospital near St. Louis. I might have married several girls to whom I had felt attracted in the university setting, but instead I finally fell in love with a beautiful woman who is a splendid wife and an excellent mother. Bette and I met in the young-adult group of the Webster Groves Presbyterian Church, where, incidentally, I was also attempting to play out a well-rehearsed yet archaic role of being in charge of the primary-grades Sunday school department, and in which I eventually and thankfully lost out to a man who was a local TV cowboy hero.

Bette at that time was the secretary to one of the Ralston Purina vice-presidents in St. Louis, having dropped out earlier from Culver-Stockton College (which I always described facetiously to our friends as a military academy in Missouri). We dated off and on for about nine months. We were married in September of 1956. I was thirty-three by this time and at last in a position to support a wife and offspring as my father had never supported my mother and me.

The next month we moved to State Hospital No. 1 in Fulton,

Missouri, where I was chief psychologist, with a joint faculty appointment at the University of Missouri. In 1960 I accepted the role of visiting professor of psychology at the University of Kansas, and the following year assumed the position of mental health consultant for the National Institute of Mental Health in the regional office in San Francisco. NIMH was, of course, charged with the responsibility of promotion of a national mental health program, with a heavy emphasis on community mental health. The overall goal was advancement of community-oriented mental health operations based on a public health tradition.

Obviously this was a full-time commitment — the region encompassed California, Washington, Oregon, Nevada, Arizona, Alaska, Hawaii, Guam, and Samoa. The outstanding virtue of the position was the involvement in the "growing edge" of everything new and progressive in mental health programs. The frustration was the limited depth of involvement — we acted largely as firemen to the urgent demands from the community and from various state programs. It was this and the large amount of time spent in traveling (I logged over 500,000 miles' flying in six years) that finally brought my wife and me to consider a university appointment. The University of Illinois seemed to offer the best possible opportunity to stop traveling and to become engaged in the training of clinical graduate students.

Recovery in a
Behavior-Oriented Environment

When I was recruited to inaugurate a program of training in community mental health at the University of Illinois, I interpreted it as an honor to be requested to return to the campus from which I had graduated seventeen years earlier, since this kind of appointment is usually considered "academic inbreeding" and is frowned upon. I came with the realization that the clinical psychology section had achieved within recent years a considerable distinction for producing students steeped in behavior therapy and practice, and I looked forward to learning more about the ways in which behavior modification might be coordinated or even integrated with community psychology. Unfortunately, the stroke intervened shortly after my return to Illinois.

Three months after the stroke, I took, very hesitantly, as my first new assignment, a course in supervising students in a practicum in psychotherapy, while I resumed working again on the community program. When I was originally hired, I was given to understand that I was to leaven a bit the strong behavioral leanings of the clinical faculty through my personal acceptance of cognitive theory, "meaning," and psychodynamics — or so I believed. As a result, in the fall of 1968 I deliberately initiated a laboratory on the hypnotherapeutic use of "unconscious symbolic productions." The content of the course was quite distant from behavior modification as it was currently being taught, but based on twenty years of experience, I really felt that I had something to offer in this area. At the very least it would be provocative and would give rise to some animated discussions which, somehow, I hoped I could handle.

In the efforts of dealing with my personal priority — rehabilitation — the fact that the majority of the staff members were dedicated to a behavior reference was a very crucial issue. As I began to recover and to resume teaching, writing, and even doing research again, I was confronted at every turn with the decided difference between the basic values of the faculty and what I had been trained in and practiced. In a very real sense, I couldn't have chosen a worse predicament than to have my stroke within weeks of coming to such an intellectually adverse environment. Plunked down among strict behavior-modificationists, I found little reinforcement for my cognitive-dynamic framework.

It wasn't that I found the staff personally vindictive in promoting their belief in social learning theory; quite the contrary, they were far too gentlemanly to pick on someone who had recently been through a CVA and was still obviously suffering from severe problems in communication. But if any changes were going to be effected, it was patently clear that the one who was going to have to change was me. At the beginning, I told myself that all of my efforts must be mobilized into the fundamental attempt to get my brain functioning again. On the other hand, emotionally, I think that I had already begun to react against this authoritarian or forced challenge and this is probably why I was secretly so perverse as even to try at all in my condition to teach a course in hypnosymbolism.

I had taught a variation of this course much earlier at the University of Missouri and the University of Kansas. In both of the previous teaching experiences, the students had been quite opposed as a body to the use of hypnosis, but more or less accepting of the psycho-analytic theory that underlay it. In the present situation, the first thing that struck me was the lack of opposition to hypnosis, but the complete disavowal of the underlying theory. I hadn't appreciated the intense behavioral bent with which the students had been imbued by the dedicated members of the clinical staff and their total rejection of any "dynamic" point of view. In short, they completely rejected the use of hypnosis to delve into the meaning of the patients' symbolic productions. In their eyes what I attempted to teach them was quite unscientific in comparison to the social learning theory which they had been taught was the *only* objective way of dealing with emotional problems. I represented to them the "old-fashioned medical modeler" point of view, i.e., a psychoanalytic practitioner.

I really was an eclectic, or, as I have learned to call it, a "synthesizer," rather than someone with a strictly psychoanalytic frame of reference. The thesis that I attempted to advance in my course was that hypnosis allows access to the symbol-translating mechanism and that some hypnotized subjects can carry interrupted dreams to completion, produce a dream as a result of direct suggestion, or even interpret dreams and other symbolic fantasies. These claims originated, of course, from Freudian theory, but my ideas differ in a great number of respects from psychoanalytic tenets. For example, while the therapist directly sets the stage through hypnosis for the production of dreaming, he exercises great care to be completely nondirective in the interpretation of the symbols produced; the patient's associations to the symbols are always radial rather than linear so they clearly relate to the here and now of current problem situations rather than back to any infantile substructure, and so forth. I realize that my particular approach may not be too distant from the practices of some ego analysts.

The attitude of behavior therapists toward hypnosis is interesting to examine. They seem to have borrowed heavily from the supposition that hypnosis is a special form of role-playing elicited solely by the demands emanating from the context and the placebo effect of the therapist. This conception of hypnosis had previously been advanced by White (1941) and Sarbin (1950), among others, and is still advanced forcefully today by Barber (1960). It appeals to the scientifically-minded by reducing the complex phenomenon to the ultimate simplicity, i.e., it all depends on the waking suggestibility of the subject. However, the majority of authorities in the area, including myself, are well aware that there exist today (as in the past) theories which are compatible with almost every known disposition, each unfettered by facts which contradict some aspect of it.[1]

[1] For this reason I eventually monitored two of my graduate students to make further investigations into the theory of hypnosis susceptibility (Olson, 1970; Tostado, 1971), both of which had negative results. Through the years there

Hence, there are certain implications in the theory of hypnosis held by the behaviorists, namely, that since hypnosis is all role-playing, they hold no confidence at all that it can be used to uncover reliably the etiological factors underlying the client's symptoms. More than that, they say that even if this were possible, "insight" would be a waste of time for the clients and themselves. The whole focus of behavior modification is to change and sustain behavior with reinforcement — changes in attitude naturally follow. Conversely, they reason that it is useless to attempt to change attitude on the pretext that alterations of behavior will follow. It simply doesn't work as most conventional therapists assume.

This position was, of course, the antithesis of what I attempted to get across in my class, namely, that there is benefit in exploring the fantasy and symbols of the patient in that they often reveal "unconsciously" held attitudes which underlie the symptoms. For the behaviorists, hypnosis is simply another device for relaxation or attention-focusing that accompanies systematic desensitization, so it is accepted without much dispute. But even in this technique they maintain that they are using relaxation rather than hypnosis because it isn't defined as "hypnosis" to the patient.

There are other illustrative differences between myself and the majority of the clinical psychology faculty. Behavior therapists, from my point of view, deal with personality as if it had no cohesion or unity. They tend to single out specific symptoms and deal with them as if they had no relationship to other facets of personality. This makes sense if one subscribes to the assumption that behavior can be altered by direct modification of specific responses, although behaviorists would maintain that "all things are related to everything else." They specify the defined behavior they wish to modify and by getting rid of the aggravating symptom, they have eliminated the neurosis (the term "neurosis" is a purely explanatory concept). Even the term "symptom" is out, since it implies a concern with root causes. It is not necessary to concern yourself with the underlying causes — the

---

have been literally tens of dozens of investigations of different theories of hypnosis, all of which turned out to be negative or contradictory. Thus I held that the various theories of hypnosis were still an open question, rather than maintaining that I or anyone else, including the behaviorists, held the solution.

behavior therapist does not concern himself with postulated intermediating processes, such as the unconscious. In essence then, in a couple of sessions, (*a*) they specify the behavior they wish to eliminate, (*b*) they emphasize the conditions under which it was established, and (*c*) they counteract the active variables that maintain the response. It is all behavior-oriented, focused strictly on the "here and now," and taking account of only purely conscious responses.

Perhaps one of the greatest practical and theoretical differences lies in the attempt of the behavior therapist to avoid any stimulation of anxiety whatever in the patient. In his mind, stimulating anxiety may cause the anxiety to generalize to neutral or even positive features in the conduct of psychotherapy. In contrast, I try to utilize anxiety, subjecting the patient to as much of it as he can stand at the moment. Anxiety is used as a motivator and catalyst for the patient. I would typically use hypnosis to delve into the predisposing trauma, to examine it, with full realization of the anxiety it might generate, and then, knowing the cause of the symptom, try to structure the situation so as to eliminate the behavior. From my point of view, of course, even dynamic psychotherapists make full use of reinforcement principles to change behavior; they simply have a great deal more information about the patient, and they apply the principles subtly and not as mechanically as do many of their behavior therapist counterparts.

Since students at Illinois are conditioned against any "dynamic" therapy by their third year in graduate school, it is no wonder that they don't place much credence in an understanding of symbolism or how one could make use of the information solicited to help the client in psychotherapy. In the formal structure of my class, I presented taped case material and the underlying rationale for an hour or two, and then selected students to present a critique of what I had done. Predictably, the students tended to reject my handling of the case and explain how they would have handled it, using standard reinforcement techniques. I was naturally disappointed in my inability to get them to consider seriously alternative ways of handling the cases. I also deliberately played down hypnosis; anyone can quickly learn the rudiments of hypnosis, but I wanted to make the students think of the underlying theory and what we were attempting to achieve through the treatment. The students were unhappy over this emphasis — they wanted to learn the skill in the technique so they might apply it to other more acceptable techniques such as their formal reinforcement schedules, Ellis's rational therapy, Lazarus's emotive therapy, modeling, the logical problem-solving approach, Salter's assertion training, labeling and expressing the effect, etc.

Despite the extensive theoretical differences, during this first attempt to teach hypnosymbolization I naturally blamed much of my inability to communicate with the students on my language disability. It was clear to me that without the brain damage I would be a much more imposing representative of the dynamic orientation than I was. Nevertheless, in teaching the course again in the 1969-70 school year, I adopted a modified strategy, showing a much greater awareness of the behavioristic predilections of my students and trying to avoid some of the more obviously semantic aspects that they were conditioned against. We were engaged in somewhat similar techniques but simply labeling them by different names and rationalizing them by different theoretical positions. The majority of students trained at Illinois are deliberately negatively conditioned to terms that smack of psychoanalysis, such as unconscious, psychodynamic, resistance, transference, projective, etc. When we finally got around to defining what was meant by our respective uses of the terms, we then discovered a remarkable degree of agreement.

There were other changes as well. Early in the repetition of the course, I gave the students a demonstration of hypnotic induction, then followed this by arranging to give them the opportunity to enter hypnosis themselves via group induction; finally, I gave each of them a chance to induce hypnosis in individual volunteers. Having been trained in behavioral psychology, they were at first very skeptical of hypnosis; however, they found all of this particularly intriguing, especially their uniform success in individual induction, which they hadn't expected but which raised many questions about the phenomenon. Finally, I requested them at least in our class time together to adhere as closely as they could to the role of a hypnotherapist in both theory and technique, as I attempted to role-play it within the context of the class, reinforcing my request by having their final grade depend in part upon their adherence. Acceptance of this approach forestalled many of the more obvious resistances that I had encountered the year before and gave them practice by immersion into what I was trying to teach them. I think that I was at least partially successful in this second attempt. I have described the experience somewhat more objectively in a journal article.[2]

The objectives of the course included the attempt to make the students aware of the necessity of looking at the human individual as a whole, of the importance of the meaning of events not overtly related to the problem behavior, and of the complexity of human behavior. The hope is that behavioral students would not be quite so disposed to dismiss quickly the reports of clients that aren't directly relevant to their preconceived notions of human behavior. The importance of symbolic generalization and association was made quite evident in my mind, and the existence and importance of these processes is a definite area that the behaviorist has not come to grips with at all.

In the final analysis, let me acknowledge the value of behavior therapy as I have been exposed to it for the past several years. I am impressed by the fact that as long as the aspects of the problem are clearly defined and where the environment of the client is open to specific control, behavior therapy seems to work. It seems clearly effective with many children, for example, where the parents and/or teacher are involved and can see that a reinforcement schedule is consistently applied. It also works with well-motivated adults who wish to alter fairly discrete symptoms and who are not resistant to the prescribed treatment and/or where the wife or husband is influential and cooperative.

I am convinced that remarkable transformations of behavior can be effected with behavior therapy within a relatively short period of time. It is an effective variation of a time-limited, brief, or crisis-oriented treatment modality — and maybe this is all that any sort of psychotherapy can purport to be. However, I was also clearly aware (as the students were not) that the clients they saw in the psychological clinic were carefully screened and selected, and that since I was employed during the summer when clinical graduate students had left, I was left to carry on with clients whose treatment could not be terminated for emotional reasons and for whatever reason had not

[2] Exposure of a "medical modeler" to behavior modification. *International Journal of Clinical and Experimental Hypnosis,* forthcoming.

responded to behavior techniques. Thus I would still maintain that in actual fact dynamic and behavior practices are quite complementary when applied to the natural spread of clients or patients requesting help.

The virtue of providing a client "insight" into how a maladjusted behavior was learned is that it provides him added motivation to change, it reduces resistances, and it provides precise information on the value of a planned behavior schedule in training him how to change in a desired direction. It is not really a question of whether attitude changes cause a change in behavior or whether an alteration in perception precedes a change in behavior; both things should go on simultaneously. I have been persuaded during the past couple of years of the benefit of getting desired behavior going and having it followed by positive consequences so that the behavior will be maintained; I hope that the social learning practitioners, in turn, will become more amenable in time to teaching clients an awareness of the antecedents as well as the consequences which dictate their behavior, without getting involved in semantic games played by the behavior modifiers.

What I have depicted here are not unemotional perceptions of the events that transpired in my early recovery. Truthfully, I cannot pick out a single faculty member with whom I had a poor relationship, but collectively they reminded me more and more of the militant chauvinism that used to typify psychoanalytic institutes twenty-five to thirty years before. I could in one sense understand the fanaticism that always comes at the beginning with any radical departure, especially one that was being promoted by psychology versus the dominant medical-psychiatric philosophies (not unlike the nondirective counseling laid down by Carl Rogers, a psychologist, in the early 1940s). As I perceived it, it was some sort of miracle that I always kept my reactions under control; on the other hand, I had no choice — because of what I had recently been through I had absolutely no confidence in causing any more than a disconcerted ripple or two. Whether or not it was correct, I had the impression that I could have recovered quicker under a more tolerant situation.

As will be related in the next chapter, when I actually became involved as a client in a form of behavior modification, it turned out *not* to be nearly as aversive as I had thought. I learned that to a large extent behavior therapists use anything and everything that might turn out to be effective and efficient, as long as they can rationalize it in their highly attenuated social learning theory.

References

Barber, T. X., and Glass, L. B. 1962. Significant factors in hypnotic behavior. *Journal of Abnormal and Social Psychology, 64,* 222-28.

Olson, R. P. 1970. The effects of motivation and expectation upon hypnotic susceptibility: a reappraisal. Unpublished Ph.D. dissertation, University of Illinois, Urbana.

Sarbin, T. R. 1950. Contributions to role-taking theory: I. Hypnotic behavior. *The Psychological Review, 57,* 255-70.

Tostado, J. A. 1971. Semantic differential differences between susceptible and nonsusceptible hypnotic subjects. Unpublished master's thesis, University of Illinois, Urbana.

White, R. W. 1941. A preface to the theory of hypnotism. *Journal of Abnormal and Social Psychology, 36,* 477-505.

8

Systematic Desensitization
WITH JAMES F. CALHOUN

I

In the months after terminating speech therapy I searched for some other type of treatment that might enable me to continue working on my remaining problems. But for one reason or another I was hesitant about some of the professional clinicians whom I knew. It is all too true that when you know psychotherapists too well, it becomes relatively easy for them to lose their placebo effects. It was probably also out of consideration for their busy schedules that I decided not to bother them. It dawned upon me finally that I would be downright foolish if, as a member of an outstanding department which specialized in training behavior modificationists, I didn't try to take advantage of the situation, even though we weren't on the best of terms theoretically.

At the beginning of the fall semester in 1969, I got the permission of a clinical faculty member to audit his course in desensitization, and after a month I approached him as a potential client, but he didn't feel that he could accept me. I continued searching, and at the beginning of the spring term I finally located a recently graduated Ph.D., Jim Calhoun, whom I had monitored in therapy and for whom I had great respect, to accept me for treatment. This chapter deals with the eleven appointments, a total of eighteen hours over a four-month period, with a behavior therapist.

The initial objective was to ascertain how much of my remaining problem was anxiety-induced, and then what, if anything, could be done about reducing the tension that I still experienced. I was aware, of course, that Gordon Paul's dissertation (1966), which gave so much impetus to systematic desensitization in this particular program, was on the treatment of anxiety in a brand of speech disorder. I was skeptical about the benefits of any form of treatment, but was thankful that the therapist would even consider working with me. Jim mentioned that, among other reasons, he personally felt that this was an opportunity to repay society partially for an excellent job therapists had done in rehabilitating his father-in-law, who had some years earlier suffered a stroke.

For those who are unfamiliar with systematic desensitization, a brief description of the technique would seem in order. Clients undergoing *relaxation training* recline comfortably in a chair, close their eyes, and listen to the therapist's calm, soft voice, repeatedly suggesting that they are becoming more and more relaxed. The client is taught to become relaxed by successively tensing and relaxing various muscle groups through the body. In behavior therapy, muscle relaxation is viewed as a means of depressing the autonomic nervous system. Physiological reactions, rather than psychological defenses, are emphasized. The client is taught to recognize and discriminate between bodily sensations associated with tension when anxiety-provoking stimuli are presented.

Treatment in systematic desensitization begins with a discussion of what makes the client anxious and from that an *anxiety hierarchy* is constructed. The items within each hierarchy are arranged in order from weakest to strongest in eliciting an anxiety response, and care is taken to space the items so as to form subjectively equal intervals. Each item or anxiety-eliciting stimulus is presented within a detailed, specific, and concrete context. New data may, of course, appear during treatment, necessitating a revision of the hierarchies.

Within *desensitization proper,* each hierarchy item is repeated at least twice, working up the hierarchy from weakest to strongest stimuli, with the therapist insuring that higher items are not presented until each lower item can be imagined without disturbance. Precise timing of the presentation is considered critical. The client is instructed to visualize a scene for ten seconds, to relax for thirty to forty-five seconds, and then, if no anxiety has been signaled, to visualize the same scene for another ten seconds. If the patient reports any anxiety to an item, he is immediately instructed to stop visualizing the scene, and relaxation is again induced. After sixty seconds of relaxation, the same item may be presented again in "diluted" form (either by shortening exposure time or by adding factors to the scene which are known to lower the intensity of the response), or a lower item from the hierarchy may be reintroduced (Paul, 1969). Each session is concluded with a "successful" item presented, so that the client may leave relaxed and feeling good. Succeeding sessions begin where previous sessions terminated, until all hierarchies have been completed. Theoretically, then, all anxiety-provoking stimuli have become associated with relaxation so that they will no longer elicit anxiety responses.

I was surprised at the first meeting when Calhoun showed up on crutches, having broken his leg trying to avoid the rush of a hostile patient. In the meeting I spelled out the nature of my problem as I saw it, and he, in turn, presented the rationale for systematic desensitization. Since he was a recent graduate from Illinois, I was frankly surprised (and pleased) at his somewhat open point of view, although it was still phrased within the behavioral framework. The gist of what we had to say was as follows:[1]

Session 1, February 28, 1970

THER.: We had better differentiate out the reality that we've got here, since it's a reality which is unlike most desensitization cases. Typically, you didn't know how to get up in front of a group and make a speech because you didn't have the appropriate skills for preparing a speech. Then it would be a matter of teaching the skills as well as desensitizing because the lack of knowledge of the skills is realistic. I can desensitize you to the conditioned anxiety associated with talking to someone because this is the anxiety that is there simply because you feel somewhat inadequate historically due to some experiences before your stroke. But we have the problem of the old conditioned anxiety plus the realistic problem of your inability to change set, to respond to questions that require some conceptualization, etc. Okay. We can desensitize you for the

[1] Every therapy session was recorded according to mutual agreement.

conditioned anxiety, and we can temporarily desensitize you to the realistic anxiety. But you'll become once again sensitized simply because the realistic problem won't go away. The reality brought on by your stroke is still there. Were I able to teach you *how* to conceptualize, that would be a different matter. Then you could actually perform the behavior and you wouldn't feel anxious. So there's that restriction that we have in that area.

The other way to go about it is not unlike Will Therapy, not unlike Rational-Emotive Therapy, to attempt to reconsider the significance, the value, the importance of being able to appropriately conceptionalize every time it's demanded. In other words, it is very important for you to be able to answer such questions, and for you to give a very reasonable conceptually sound and concise answer. In other words, to look good in every situation. What I'm saying is that if we can't rapidly retrain you to conceptualize or write rapidly, then we can reevaluate the situation which causes the anxiety — let's look at your perception of reality and perhaps change some of the importance of certain aspects of it. In other words, maybe it isn't *that* important to give a concise, conceptual answer to a student when he asks it, in which case what we're doing is changing the reality or your perception of reality in that situation. So what had previously been a source of realistic anxiety no longer is, in which case we can desensitize you to the conditioned anxiety, change your perception of the realistic anxiety, and hence not have it resensitize you. You see then we have a two-edged sword that we're working with: one is the conditioned anxiety which we can take care of, the other is the realistic anxiety which we are handling through having you change the reality. Ellis would say "what difference does it make if you can't give the concise, conceptual answer!"[2] What's going to happen? A student won't get up and walk out of the class. This is the kind of approach we would have to take in dealing with that reality.

Moss: I don't think the students would demand a highly conceptual answer from me, but I would. I would demand this of myself.

Ther.: That's exactly what I'm saying. What I'm asking you to do

[2] Albert Ellis, the originator of rational-emotive therapy, whom I discovered was acceptable to behavior therapists at Illinois.

is to reevaluate the significance or importance in terms of your value of what you place on it.

Moss: This sort of thing has been said to me often before, by my wife and others. And I realize this would be difficult to do because what we are actually attacking is my whole style of life, my whole professional life-style.

Ther.: I'm saying this with the realization that you perceive most of us as behaviorists and what I am saying really isn't what a behaviorist would do. I'm talking like a Rogerian or an Ellison. But the fact of the matter is that how you perceive the situation is how you are going to respond to it.

Moss: This is the whole essence of therapy that I have espoused for years. If you can change the perception of the problem, then you have changed the problem in reality.

Ther.: And what I am going to ask you to do is to discover the consequences of your performing certain acts that imply you do not feel it is all that important. . . . Now, the theory of relaxation is a package composed of three parts: relaxation training, the anxiety hierarchy, and desensitization proper. We have already talked about the hierarchy in defining demonstrable situations which are progressively anxiety-stimulating and you will be asked to imagine these anxiety-provoking situations. The real active factor is desensitization, which is relaxation. It is a skill which can be learned. It is not hypnosis; hypnosis is passive while this calls for active participation. [This is a distinction that I still can't buy today. *C.S.M.*] It comes from Jacobson at the University of Chicago in the early thirties where he found that if a person is muscularly relaxed, then all of the autonomic areas are also relaxed.[3] This is an assumption that has always been made, there's no real documented evidence to show why this occurs. There's no real theory as to why it happens, but it does — there is a great deal of clinical and experimental evidence which demonstrates this.

[3] Relaxation training began with Edmund Jacobson, a physiologist, who developed a physiological method of combating tension and anxiety. He discovered that by systematically tensing and releasing various muscle groups and by learning to discriminate the resulting sensations, it is possible for a person to experience a feeling of deep relaxation. He published the results in *Progressive Relaxation,* 1929.

The principle is ridiculously simple: when you tense the muscles, the muscle potential rises, and if you let go suddenly, then the muscle falls below the adaptation level, which causes the clinical effect. If the muscle is not tensed following that, it will stay below and actually seek a new adaptation level. So what the relaxation procedure involves is tensing and then releasing all the muscles of the body, with the consequence that all muscles will be below the adaptation level and very relaxed. We'll practice this and then eventually I'll give you the prescription to go out and practice this twice a day during the week. This will require you to wear comfortable clothes, take off your shoes, and relax in a comfortable chair. We want to continue relaxation training until you can relax by recall so that you'll be able to relax yourself on cue [or auto-hypnosis?].

As my first "homework" assignment, I was to try to discriminate the specific, concrete interpersonal events that triggered off my anxiety, which of course meant practically anything relating to any human contact where I was to verbalize. In short, my treatment proceeded along more or less standard behavioral lines for the first half-dozen sessions. The second session began with the six items that I had produced in the interim. These items began at near zero anxiety and proceeded up to, but not including, the anxiety felt during interprofessional contacts. However, the therapist immediately pointed out reservations, stating that among other things, they were much too wordy, not specific enough to visualize nor concrete enough, and not as close together in terms of anxiety as he would like. I present here the six items for the reader to inspect; they can be contrasted with the twenty-five items listed in Table 1.

1. Watching television is probably the least anxiety-arousing activity. TV allows one to be an observer without actually partaking of the actual interpersonal relationship. Once in a while when watching TV, I engage in a fantasy, telling myself that the "accident" never happened or that I am fully recovered, but then I am brought back to reality by the next contact I make. When I am more "reality oriented," I sometimes listen to what a person is saying — usually this occurs on a news program like the "Today" show — and I marvel at the complicated way a person has of talking without essentially any awareness of the complexity of translating thought into language.

2. I would place my relationship with my two youngest children (Kevin, age seven, and Julie, age nine) at the lowest anxiety-arousing level. We frequently play where verbalizations are at a minimum, and even where they are not, I still have enough confidence to believe that my verbal facility will make me understood. And even when I make a mistake, like calling them by the wrong name, I know the children know about my "accident" and will tend to laugh about the errors. For instance, playing tag with them about the house, teaching Julie her multiplication tables, or lying down in bed with Kevin or Julie at the end of the day and seriously attempting to explain something to them, usually something about relating to others.

3. With Joel, our oldest boy, age twelve, the relationship is getting somewhat more complicated. He is a "big" twelve and fairly intelligent. I find it more difficult to engage him in rational discussion, especially because he is old enough to begin having sparks of independence. For example, we are continually trying to get him to dress warmly enough when he goes outside in brisk weather. A more complicated example was when Joel was a patrol guard last year and found that some of the black children disregarded the guards' commands and then in some instances actually threw rocks at them. Joel tended to respond with aggression toward the Negroes rather than taking his complaint to the principal or the supervising teacher. When confronted with his behavior he maintained that it never did any good to bring his complaints to the teacher. We talked about this several times, but don't feel that we made much of an inroad. I am hesitant about discussing such things with him and prefer, if possible, to leave it to my wife, because I know the situation is complicated and also involves some emotion, both of which get in the way of my language formation.

4. With my wife I talk about anything and everything, although the complexity of the topic gives me some hesitation now and then. We often talk about my condition and our future, and my mood swings between being relatively optimistic or occasionally highly pessimistic. Most of our conversations are in private; as a result I occasionally let myself regress and don't think through before speaking. There is a tendency to leave the disciplining of the children to my wife, rather than having to talk it through with everyone; yet I am not really completely satisfied with her activity, since it impresses me that she isn't firm enough and her actions lack consistency. But all in all I feel very comfortable in discussing matters with her privately.

5. With my mother or father-in-law, I am again relatively relaxed,

but not as much as with my own family members. Much of what we talk about is rather mundane, but let the conversation drift to, say, a passing news item, and chances are I will begin to feel mild anxiety. As soon as the topic shifts to something remote from my everyday life, the possibility increases that I will flounder in finding the correct word to express a particular feeling or thought. For example, when my father-in-law, who is rather rigid and highly conservative, says something about his own personal views, I don't tend to respond, first because of the courtesy that I feel I owe him, but second because it would necessitate my calling forth words which I am not sure I could marshal. And the same goes for my mother, although usually, in relation to her, I will take issue but again rather quickly retire into myself.

6. When a neighbor enters the picture, then for the first time I clam up; even if it is a neighbor that I know well, and we just chance to meet, I am immediately on my guard, carefully weighing every utterance. For example, when we replaced our regular logs with a gas log and this topic came up in conversation with a neighbor, I suddenly couldn't remember the name of the substitute. As a result I am always thinking how to end the interaction as soon as possible. If the neighbor has something to talk to me about, like should we put up a joint fence, then I have to fight against panic. I simply can't engage in social chit-chat the way I did once. It is interesting that over the phone I must sound (nearly) normal, but I can't carry this role off in any face-to-face confrontation.

The second part of the interview that day dealt with my training in the relaxation of sixteen muscle groups, beginning with the right hand and forearm and stopping with my left foot. My tensing and releasing the various muscles was enhanced by the quiet verbal stimulation of the therapist. By the end of the session, the feeling of relaxation was pronounced, although I would still maintain that it was very similar to hypnosis. I was told that I should go home and practice relaxation twice a day at least, but also was cautioned not to make the sessions closer than three hours apart. To paraphrase William James in his comments about Christian Science, I wasn't sure what this would do for my aphasia, but I was fairly certain that I would probably die happier because of it.

In the ensuing three sessions, the six items were refined into very specific concrete and replicable statements that were interactive and constructive; and the relaxation was focused on the hierarchy listed in Table 1 that was constructed from them. I had progressed sufficiently on the relaxation training so that the sixteen muscle groups were combined into seven and then four wholesale groupings in anticipation of the time when I would suspend practice and need only "think of relaxation" by remembering what the sensations were like, to get my body instantly and completely relaxed in any stress situation.

TABLE 1. THE ORDERING OF MY ANXIETY HIERARCHY

Low

1. Watching television and being caught up in what's happening on the screen.
2. Playing tag about the house with Kevin and/or Julie.
3. Sitting silently and telling myself that the "accident" had never happened or that I was now fully recovered.

Moderate

4. Marveling at the way a person interviewed on a TV newscast spoke spontaneously without an apparent thought as to how his thinking was translated into language.
5. Teaching Julie her multiplication tables.
6. Having to explain to Julie or Kevin the implications of something serious, e.g., Kevin being distractible in school or overly aggressive.
7. A serious discussion with Joel, e.g., the Arab-Israeli controversy, or being a school guard and the differences with Negro kids.
8. A discussion with my wife about our future, e.g., whether we should consider another kind of position for me (the problem of my past record versus what I can do now).

Medium

9. Interaction with my mother or my father-in-law about trivial or more important things, either of which is anxiety-arousing if I have to assume initiative in the conversation.
10. Interaction with a neighbor, even around mundane topics, such as replacing our regular fire logs with gas logs.
11. Contact with a neighbor who has something important to talk with me about, e.g., putting up a joint fence.
12. Individual contacts with students in the hall to talk about incidental things.
13. Daily contact with any of the secretaries to talk about anything.
14. A meeting to talk privately with either Julian, Don Peterson, or Doug.
15. These therapy sessions (general).

High

16. A meeting with individual students about monitoring them on a case.
17. A lecture before a group where I had detailed notes on my presentation.
18. The same thing except with additional time given to questions-and-answers.
19. An invitation for Bette and me to a faculty or neighborhood party.
20. An invitation for dinner.
21. Our own party or dinner (I as host).

Very High

22. A seminar rather than a didactic lecture — with a good deal of time spent in spontaneous give-and-take.
23. A staff meeting where I don't have any notes but am called upon to speak.
24. A staff meeting where I know some of the items to be discussed and I have prepared notes.
25. A staff meeting where I don't have notes but must volunteer information at some length, e.g., some matter of policy about CMH.

I was, of course, keeping a log on my reactions to behavior therapy, and at this time noted that I was going along with the technique out of sheer desperation, but that "I'll be darned if I can believe it will work." There were a number of reasons for my skepticism other than learning-theory rationale that stood behind the treatment. First of all, I didn't believe that I was that sensitive in differentiating feelings of anxiety in reference to the individual items. I really could not determine in many instances that one item was any more or less anxiety-arousing than another; and if I, a relatively sophisticated psychologist, couldn't discriminate, how in the world could the usual neurotic client distinguish each item in terms of the anxiety potential, especially when care was taken to space the items so as to form subjectively equal intervals? Then when we got into the desensitizing procedure itself, I found myself having to signal anxiety as the items progressed, then indicating that after two or three times the feeling had dissipated — all of it predicated on the expectations of the therapist rather than the fact that I did or did not actually experience any anxiety. In this sense, I was role-playing in terms of the placebo of therapeutic context and was very much aware of it, although I expect that a more naive person might not have been. The process of relaxation intrigued me, however; it reminded me vaguely of the feeling after orgasm, when any movement or even thinking threatens to disequilibrate the chemical sensation of total relaxation. This is the reason I always resented having to respond to the therapist, for example, even to indicate that one muscle group was as relaxed as the previous muscle group, etc.

Despite my uncertainty about the desensitization aspects of therapy, it did seem that over these weeks I became a little less anxious and a little more secure. The rationale presented by the therapist that "we are undermining a building (i.e., anxiety) from the bottom, and as each floor is eaten away it drops down, and what was originally twenty stories is now only ten in terms of the anxiety level that it arouses" wasn't convincing to me, but some of the discussions that we engaged in were. He felt, for instance, that it was important that I stop apologizing for my alleged weakness.

THER.: I have noticed a significant improvement in your conversation just since we have been meeting. Your conversations have changed noticeably. You are much more free, open, and relaxed. You don't even appear anxious to me in your external appearance, only in the content of what you say. Motorically you don't show it at all. This is why I place such emphasis on the feedback you give yourself and not so much on what others give you.

Moss: In other words, if I didn't open my mouth and say something about how I felt, they would never know. They would be deluded into thinking that I felt very comfortable. And yet I feel compelled to share with people the fact that I feel very uncomfortable.

THER.: I think this is one of the Freudian defense mechanisms, that by telling others you have protected yourself against evaluation. Try not to tell people exactly what you feel — otherwise they would never know. Stop apologizing! Stop telling people that you are not nearly as well as you appear. Stop being self-depreciatory. Every time you make a mistake, you're going to resensitize yourself. It is all relative. You will still have a fear of its recurring even though we have reduced the degree. It all resides in your self-labeling. Your goal should not be zero, to be flawless, that is the crux. At some point you're going to have to accept more flaws than previously. But the goal should be in not apologizing. Simply accept your mistake and take it as a matter of course. Don't focus on the mistake and draw attention to it by apologizing.

Moss: When I make a mistake I should learn how to whistle Dixie! Why can't I behave as I did previously — it is utter nonsense that I can't.

Ther.: Don't allow yourself to get bent out of shape over this!

The thing that triggered off this discussion was my decision to go to California for a job interview. I had toyed around with accepting a position within the V.A. as researcher, but for a number of reasons decided against it. Then the possibility of a job as a chief psychologist in a federal prison presented itself (p. 169) and I decided to interview for the job. To make an abbreviated story out of a long and anxiety-filled decision, my wife and I went to visit after the fourth session with Jim Calhoun, came back for the fifth session with the report that the trip was delightful, that everything had gone quite well, even though it had been frantic. I was acceptable to the warden and to Washington, and now I was confronted with having to make a final decision. The following week I decided to take the position and told Don Peterson and Mort Weir. I think that out of the experience I learned that my functioning was about as good as it needed to be, while still recognizing that by my former standards it left something to be desired (but emphasizing that no one knew this except myself or possibly former colleagues who might note the difference).

Session 5, April 4, 1970

Ther.: [in response to my telling him the story about the job interview]: I still hear you saying that you maybe fooled the people in the amount that you communicated with them — when you actually get out there they are going to find out about you.

Moss: I may be saying that I am actually fooling myself — that I can make this jump.

Ther.: Yes, you may not be giving yourself credit. Don't build it into a full-blown phobia. You have given it a great deal of consideration.

Moss: But there are so many people that depend on me — my wife, my three children, my mother, even my father-in-law. I would

hate to think that I was misleading all of them by my decision
to switch jobs.

THER.: Are they that totally dependent upon you? Where do you
draw the line? There is a degree of risk even in staying here, but now
that you are making a decision, you have given up one risk for
another, but the world isn't going to collapse about your ears even
if this doesn't work out the way you expect. In a sense you expect
it to collapse, but the world isn't going to stop. You're putting too
much finality on the one decision. It is important but not *that*
important.

MOSS: I am sure the world will go on, but I'm not at all certain
that I could abide by it.

THER.: Let's keep the decision in perspective — don't build up the
situation so it is more important than it is.

MOSS: It's hard to do in such crucial decision-making. Before this
accident I could do or be almost anything I put my mind to, but
following this stroke came a necessary readjustment, so that now
I'm taking a much lower position than what I thought possible three
years ago. I'm moving several steps down. I hate to think of what
the next job will be if I fail this one.

THER.: It's a very unpleasant thought even to consider, and moving
backwards is a rough experience. To be behavioral for the moment,
all of the rewards and the reinforcers that you had previously
received before your accident to keep you going are —

MOSS: Washed out!

THER.: Exactly, and now you have to start over again.

MOSS: And that's very hard to accept! I realize that intellectually
you are correct — even this job may be too hard. But I don't know
if this comes about, how then I will adjust. It isn't the reward and
prestige of the job, rather it boils down to the security that I can
give my family.

THER.: You need to recognize that there are other places even after
this, and secondly, I am not all that convinced that you are fooling
them that much. From your perception you are making too great
a contrast between what you think you can do now and what you
did before, and you are projecting the contrast onto them.

MOSS: But if they don't really know me — if all they have to go on is my *vita*. I think they are thinking of me in terms of that piece of paper rather than knowing what I am now or what I can actually do. I have told everyone that I have suffered a stroke and I do try to spell out the residuals.

THER.: But you give no hint of your word-finding difficulties, especially in conversations which you have prepared. You give an occasional slip, but to you knowing that you didn't do this previously, it is a tragic error, but it's not that frequent. But to you, knowing what a struggle it is to talk and to be aware and alert, and also feeling very, very bad when you are stuck for a word, I can empathize with you.

I wonder if, in a conversation, what would happen if you focused on the 90 percent of the time that you do find the correct word instead of the 10 percent that you don't?

Moss: You are correct, it is always the latter that comes back to me — which in turn comes back to the fact that I have always been highly perfectionistic in anything I do. And 10 or even 5 percent is too much. It is just the fact that now it happens much more frequently to me — I have never really accepted the fact that I can't accomplish what I did before.

THER.: And I'm saying that in their perceptions, 90 percent is excellent! I want you to keep meditating on this and not to forget this. Maybe you should program yourself to focus on the 90 percent. As long as you continue to project your perception onto them, then you'll never see yourself as doing well. As long as you continue to do this you're going to be miserable; you'll be hypersensitive to their reactions to you. We can get you relaxed and desensitized but over and above that we also want to get you feeling satisfied and somewhat happy.

Moss: And in my present frame of mind, I don't think I'll ever be happy again.

THER.: You're not too old a dog to be taught a new trick or two.

Moss: But the perfectionism goes so far back, I don't even know where it began. Somehow I was taught this even in childhood — that unless I phrase things very effectively and explicitly, people won't listen. I really don't think that people listen very much to anyone; most of the time is spent on their own thoughts. I think this is the truth, and I learned very young that I must say things very directly and concisely and explicitly and then shut up. There were people who commented on the fact that I always had such excellent command, such facility to express my own thoughts. Even in our conversations there is a quality that reflects this point.

THER.: I think you are very right and what I am asking you is to give up these strongly held beliefs and to substitute other beliefs in their place. This is something that really follows relaxation and desensitization. Give yourself a fair shake — 90 percent is pretty good for anybody.

Moss: I realize what you are saying, and it would be nice if I could modify what has become for me a whole style of relating to other people, but it is such a well-learned habit, I don't know what I can substitute for it.

THER.: Initially, I want you to praise yourself for communicating appropriately a fair proportion of the time.

Moss: As a matter of fact, thinking about our communication this hour, I am relatively well satisfied.

THER.: I am too.

Moss: I don't know what makes me effective one time and have a loss of effectiveness other times.

THER.: Try to focus more on the times that you are satisfied.

Moss: You are correct, I don't attend to conversations that go well — only to those that don't.

THER.: It's kind of like trying to teach the parents to praise children. Parents often say, "But children are supposed to be good, it's only when they are bad that we attend to them." We all develop expectancies. When things go well, then we don't have to attend to them.

Moss: That analogy makes some sense to me.

II

In the seventh session, I took some pains to point out tactfully what some of my objections were to continuing on with the sessions structured primarily about systematic desensitization. Even though we were only halfway through the anxiety hierarchy, it apparently struck a responsive chord within the therapist, possibly because of the passage of time and because his schedule made it necessary to make more headway before the interviews were concluded. The following session is reported almost in its entirety and is followed by the highlights of the remaining four treatment interviews. The essence of these sessions deals basically with tactics designed to alter my perception of my CVA and the residual qualities which affected my performance.

Session 7, April 18, 1970

THER.: Have you been communicating your decision to people?

Moss: Yes, Don announced it to the staff Wednesday, so little by little things are taking shape. We are working on selling the house and a "For Sale" sign should go up in a day or two.

THER.: Well, good. I imagine it is keeping you busy now.

Moss: Yes, although, believe it or not, I am always busy. This means ordering the priorities a little differently.

THER.: Yes, real good. Did you get a chance to work on what we sort of ended with last time — working up to the actual experience of talking to somebody?

Moss: Yes, I believe so, but let's preface it a little bit. We were talking about my attempting to have a positive interpretation instead of a negative interpretation of what I do and the experiences I've had and so on. Regardless of what I do professionally or otherwise, it all adds up to a form of self-therapy. Anyway, taking the viewpoint of myself as a patient or client, somebody who must engage in continuous remediation rather than functioning as a professional person, then, in a sense, I can let myself off the hook. There were many times this week when I had a contact and after it was over I would take some pride in the way I had handled it *as an aphasic,* rather than a professional person. If I used a professional person as my standard, I think I would always have fallen short of what I think I should do. On the other hand, if I look at myself as an aphasic or as an aphasic in some sort of remission or recovery with aphasia, then I can be much more relaxed as to how I judge myself. And from that point of view, I think I had a number of positive experiences, although I did fall down a couple of times.

THER.: And you apologized?

Moss: Yes, and I could have kicked myself, but I did it just out of force of habit; but the point is that I am increasingly aware of when I do it, and if I just can remember to look at myself as a person who is engaging in self-help, rather than engaging in professional activity, this sort of gives me an "out." I don't know how long I can continue to do that but I think it does sort of let up on the pressure that I have placed myself under.

Ther.: I think one thing, that I wouldn't draw this discrimination too fine between being in constant therapy and being a professional, because I think one of the functions of our profession is that it is a combination. I've never been able to discriminate completely the fact that whenever I am doing anything, it is not only a form of benefit for someone else but a form of self-benefit. To me it is a constant interplay between the two and I would be a little hesitant in making the discrimination all that sharp.

Moss: Yes, I would agree with you but I think that prior to my cerebral insult, I, too, could look on what we were doing professionally as a form of self-help, but this was at an intellectual level. Now it is largely at the gut level and I would say at that point I almost have to make a distinction to give myself an "out."

Ther.: I understand — it is different. I am talking in terms of mine as a lot more intellectual.

Moss: Yes, and I could do that, too — two and a half years ago. That's what I am alluding to, that at some point I must reassemble or amalgamate or — I'm searching for a word — get these two points of view back together again.

Ther.: Yes, what I am wondering, would it be good if we thought about how to fade; in other words, I'm sure that the two are not total dichotomies. I'm thinking that it would be good if we considered how we could shift gently or slowly or gradually from one to the other rather than just an abrupt transition. It's like working through a desensitization hierarchy rather than simply shifting over; because you do feel more comfortable in the role as a person with a cerebral accident. To make that transition I think we can make it gradually.

Moss: I'll keep that in mind. In a way, there is something else that I don't think I have said before. When I had this accident and ever since the accident, the effects or the residual of the trauma have almost completely engulfed me. Now that doesn't really say what I mean but, time and time again, I have uppermost in my mind, "What has the effect of this been on me?" And this almost completely overshadows everything else. I'm not sure what I'm leading up to but I always felt that if I could find a therapist who would just listen to me talk about reactions from my illness, the reaction of various residuals and so on, that in a sense this would be a very great relief. Interestingly enough, I have never found such a person, or let's say that the type of person I thought I was looking for would be more of a conventional therapist. At that juncture I think that my criticality about therapists came to the fore and that there simply wasn't that type of person in the immediate vicinity.

I'm not sure what I am looking for really, but remember I told you and you read something in my autobiography about the contacts I've had with various therapists — (pause). Maybe I should start again, the contact I have had with professional people has been around — they were interested in diagnosis or assessment of me, and many of them, having gotten a diagnosis, were through with their professional responsibility. This is particularly true of medical people. But, even then, I had a couple of sessions with a therapist at Michael Reese and I had an extended period of time with several therapists over at Speech and Hearing, but each of these left me unsatisfied. Each of them had various things which they attempted to do for me and I always wanted to speak up and say, though I never did, "I want instead to spend some time dwelling on the accident itself." I don't know what the point is now in bringing it up because you, too, are engaging in what you know best and I think you are partially convinced that what you are doing may be of benefit to me. I realize that there may be considerable doubt whether this does any good for this particular type of case, but I just have a need to say that for whatever reason, the accident has completely preoccupied me, from the time it happened until now.

Let me go back and put in the perspective a little bit. When I saw Joe Wepman, I think I indicated in my sketch that he had not seen my medical records and he simply assumed that I had a very temporary block in the carotid artery and that it had been dissipated.

He said, in effect, that if it had remained in place, "you'd be a vegetable," because the brain itself couldn't exist for more than three or four minutes without oxygen. And I think later on I talked more with the medical people who had made the diagnosis and eventually discovered that it had not — the clot had not passed through the artery but instead had stopped in the inner carotid. But, anyway, in my talking with Wepman, he assured me that at the moment I had some signs of organicity; however, he said that in time I would get over these and eventually I would forget about the trauma and simply become concerned with other people and other things once more. In effect, I don't find that this has happened even yet. He thought it would happen in a matter of months, and (pause) — now I'm stuck — not stuck for words but for what is the implication of what I'm telling you.

THER.: Well, that you are still concerned about it.

Moss: Yes, but I don't know what, if anything, I expected you to do in regard to this, but somehow in the back of my mind was always the fact, because I was preoccupied with it, that given the chance to ventilate and talk about it at great length, eventually I would be over it — I would stop being preoccupied with the accident and begin to take a much more objective attitude toward other problems than myself. I don't know whether that makes sense, but I had a need to say it.

THER.: I'm trying to understand how talking about the problem, the event, would have the effect of doing that. The behaviorist would say that to dwell on the past event and to respond about it is only to reinforce the meditation about the event. And so to focus on *other* than the event, and to reinforce *that,* something that is incompatible to that, would be much more beneficial and therapeutic.

Moss: Right, O.K. I guess two points of view come to mind when you say that and I realize why you are saying this from this particular orientation. I remember a long time ago when I read Theodore Reik and there was one book, *Listening with the Third Ear.* I may have it still, I'm not sure. He said that people who are dreadfully anxious try to avoid talking about whatever subject they may be anxiety-prone about. And his point was that to attempt to forget or repress this information makes common sense, but he found through years and years that you first have to remember the event in detail, and when you remember the event, then it will automatically be forgotten. Well, this is what did make sense to me and which I had attempted to practice for years, and I thought quite successfully until now.

On top of that, the second point is that each person, when he has a trauma, reacts to it in terms of his defenses. And what I found out was that I reacted to my cerebral accident as a researcher, an experimenter. And I think I have always used this in relation to my accident, that in a sense I have tried to take an objective point of view toward my accident. And when I viewed what had happened to me, I never, hardly ever, let emotion get through or away from me. Do you see?

THER.: Yes, in other words, you did very rationally, very objectively, very matter-of-factly state that your referral to it as a cerebral accident was a constant — yes, I get this, you haven't let yourself react emotionally to it.

MOSS: So what I am saying, I guess, is that these two issues, the fact that one must first react to the trauma before he can forget it, and, secondly, the fact that obviously I have reacted as an experimenter, researcher, or whatever about my trauma — these two things seem to add up to me to the fact that maybe this is the reason why, after almost two and a half or three years, I am still almost utterly preoccupied with the results of the accident. Whether it makes any sense or not, this is what I think.

THER.: O.K. Fine. I think, well, I have some thoughts on it, but let me look at something else now. When we initially started a couple of months ago, your feeling was that we wanted to focus on the residuals of the accident in terms of your communicating with other people and reducing the frequency of blocking on words; in other words, lowering the level of anxiety and being able to communicate with the minimum amount of blocking. I don't know, but I kind of feel that I am hearing you say now that you are kind of questioning that assumption and beyond that you are saying that perhaps it is this constant preoccupation and sort of unresolved emotional reaction to the accident itself that may be also maintaining this problem.

Moss: I think both are correct. The way we originally structured the problem, I think whether I realized it or not, I was attempting to structure it in terms of how a behavior therapist would accept the problem, how I would voice it to you. And at this juncture I still say that far and away my greatest need is to be able to communicate with others and to find words to go into this communication with others. But what I am now doing is simply giving you what I think may be a broader definition of what is really wrong with me; how we originally structured it still is very paramount but I think that this is somehow related to accomplishing the original task.

Ther.: I got you. In other words, if we don't also really consider the initial emotional reaction that it will always be a source of resensitizing you or still maintaining some anxiety in the situation. It is sort of always there and always a reminder and always a cause for concern.

Moss: We got to this, my formulation of what I think is somewhat the problem at the deeper level, by your telling me that I should try to decrease the negative impression of what I was doing and try to increase the positive. That led me to think, well, I must stop really being professional.

Ther.: Go on, I think I understand.

Moss: It's only that I have reinterpreted what I am doing. I've sort of been pursuing a secret agenda — the reinterpretation between us of what I am doing. So I think that in fact we had originally determined that somehow or other I must have a reconception of what I was doing, and I automatically turned to thinking of myself as sort of being a client or patient with aphasia rather than as a professional person, and this allowed me then to reduce the exaggerated expectations I held for myself. But this in turn led me to —

Ther.: To realizing the preoccupation of the consequence. O.K. Good. I got you. So we have two things: one is to reduce the initial cause for preoccupation, the emotional response to the trauma itself *and* to reduce the maintaining or continual response to the accident, which is the blocking. In other words, every time you block, you are reminded of the accident.

Moss: Yes, and because I block almost all the time, then I am always reminded of what happened.

THER.: Therefore, it is a continual preoccupation which leads back to the initial event. In reconceptualizing what you are saying, let's use the word "catharsis" as an emotional outpouring or an emotional response. It occurred to me that implosion therapy, which is a very carthartic experience where the person is encouraged to make the focus on the anxiety or problem situation in great detail, to experience all the emotional reactions that are associated with the event, even to the point of unpleasantness, a good deal of unpleasantness —

MOSS: Yes, I think if I may say that one of my main objections to behavioral therapy, as it is practiced around here ordinarily, is, I think you — this is the hard thing to say because I don't want you to feel that I am attacking you, but in essence I have to say this to make a point — I feel again and again, regardless of whom they are seeing and what they are doing, they are entirely too cautious of any anxiety they may call forth in a patient, and as soon as they call forth any anxiety it seems to me they very quickly cut it off, or detour or bring up another point. This to me is entirely contrary to what I have always thought and believed was effective in psychotherapy. In other words, in dealing with patients and clients through twenty years, I always subjected the client to as much anxiety as I thought he could stand at the moment. If I thought there was too much anxiety, I would engage in various devices to bring it back to a level he could handle. But to me it is nonsense to bring this up even, because I don't see how you can deal with it.

THER.: What I'm saying, what I am considering at this point is that desensitization is a therapy device whereby the anxious associations in the situation are eliminated before they are able to arise and gradually increase up to where they never get to occur. Implosion is just the opposite, where you are actually eliciting it. In fact, it is the extreme opposite, because not only are you eliciting it but you are banging on it, pounding on it and telling the person suffer, suffer, suffer — experience it to its fullest extent, be miserable.

MOSS: Then in a sense implosion therapy is more akin to what I've practiced for years than is straight behavioral modification.

THER.: The reason why I bring that up is that implosion, if we do it, will be a unique application of it, similar to what we have been using in desensitization because we are asking you to "implode" a past event, something that we hope won't reoccur. And what we are saying is that we want to fully experience the emotional reaction to the situation that has occurred once, and will not reoccur, or do we want it to occur? And usually this is done in a situation where a person has a phobia problem and he has experienced it and he will probably not experience it again. But the other thing I like about implosion is that it is hard on a person for a short period of time, but, unlike traditional psychotherapy, it doesn't take as long, and we have a time problem which is relevant to both of us because I am not sure as to my availability this summer. So I'm thinking that if we do take this route, I would consider this to be a therapeutic approach to do this. In a way, I am sort of asking your reaction.

Moss: Now you said several things. You are asking my reaction to the idea itself?

Ther.: The idea of using implosion to tackle this aspect of the situation, how would you feel?

Moss: Well, I would say that I'm in favor of it, by all means. That to continue to do what we were attempting to do would take an extraordinarily long period of time. It is correct that in any or every contact I've had difficulty in finding the words that I want to use to express how I feel. And in the way we are going about it, little by little it is becoming apparent to me that we have to begin far back, very early, and I think it would take an extraordinary amount of time to ever get us around to really resolving the phobia or the anxiety that I feel.

Ther.: Great. I think you have a point. I'm recalling an article I read not too many months ago. I forget exactly what the circumstance was, but where there was a very wide range of anxiety-producing situations and had it been approached strictly from a desensitizing to those particular situations it would have taken many, many months to cover all the possibilities, whereas it was suggesting an underlying basis similar to your situation. In tackling that, rather than the actual symptomatic behaviors, it's getting rather close to the old "medical model," but I think we ought not to throw the baby out with the bath. — O.K. I buy this and I think this would be certainly something to do. Now let's go back to considering what this means. When you say your response to the accident, you got little response — I'm not sure I'm making myself clear. You said there was at one time in talking to this one doctor — that you did experience the feelings that you felt about the accident at a gut level, that you were beginning to feel. What kinds of things were you talking about, what kinds of things were you recalling? What were you thinking about? Were they implications of the accident itself? Or what?

Moss: I'm not sure what she [i.e. Doris Gruenewald] had in mind, but she attempted to structure with me, under hypnosis, a sort of forced-fantasy technique. She simply had me think back and remember what it was like in California before I moved here. In forced-fantasy technique there is sort of a projective technique, insofar as a therapist can, he or she gives the client or patient the responsibility for forming the fantasy. So she simply said, "I want you to think about anything back in California." And I fantasized that my wife and I were working out in the garden in front of the house and all of a sudden I became very tearful. And the therapist asked why was I reacting this way, and the things this brought to mind were that I had persuaded Bette to give up California, a very lovely area, and the many friends she had and a lovely home and come here. It was based almost exclusively on the fact that I felt it was time to go back into the academic world and share with people what I knew about community mental health. We had looked at a number of academic positions and I was persuaded that perhaps this was the best one available to me at the moment. In addition it was sort of an honor to be asked back to your own university. But all of a sudden it came upon me how very much I had asked her to give up, only to come back within a short period of time and experience a stroke.

Ther.:   Failing her.

Moss: Yes. And once this happened, then everything I used to persuade her to come, which was all academic on the basis that in time I would establish myself as — I'm stuck, I think I'm stuck, not because there aren't words but because I don't know what words to use, the same thing, you see. I'll stop and start again. But when I suffered the stroke then the only real reason for our coming here was lost, there was no other reason.

The fact that I had failed just completely overwhelmed me. And I began then to cry and tear up. And it went on at least for half an hour. Anyway that experience and the reaction to that experience in the next day or two led to this insight that I had really reacted to my trauma as an experimenter rather than a human being who had suffered a near-fatal trauma.

THER.: O.K. I guess what it sounds like — you had for the first time stopped and started thinking about the consequences, the real significance of the accident as far as you, professionally, as a husband, a provider, and the human in everything else that is involved — it was at that point that it hit you. Now you say that you feel that there are still things that you have not considered, you really hadn't experienced the gut level significance of it.

Moss: I think I have experienced these things intellectually.

THER.: But not at the gut level. I think what we would probably do, and this would be a little different than the regular implosion, but I think the way I would go about it would be to relax you, to have it so you could focus an image, imagine a low level of sensory input, and then I think we would take the same initial tack as she provided. Have you fantasize the "before" and I think that we would have you start considering the consequences, the implications of the accident. And carry that on for about an hour and then stop and try to keep note of what things would still be carried on. I'm saying that we can either break this up into hour segments, and it would be carried on into three or four sessions or have one long one. I think with the first one it would be good to stop after an hour so we could consider where we were. I would have you do this in a relaxed state where you could focus and tend primarily to the experience. I'm wondering — I'm not — it's going to take an awful lot, it's going to be primarily your job to cue yourself initially to the appropriate scenes, to solicit this. The difference is that implosion therapists take the prime responsibility for providing these scenes and initially you are going to have to do that because with you the cues are vague enough and I don't think I could.

Moss: I was just about to say I don't know where we would go and I don't mind this, in fact, I think it is preferable that I don't know where we would go. I hate to complicate the situation even more but, in a sense, now I may be wrong on this, I maintained during these two and a half years, a very nice equilibrium. I haven't felt depressed and whenever I encountered trauma, I have always been able to look at things in a very objective fashion. What I am saying is maybe that when we work through this defense as I call it, I might become really depressed. I don't know, perhaps it isn't really my nature to be depressed — I have never really been depressed in my whole life. The only reason that I say this is that I have surmounted this accident in a relatively stable way, I think, and this is in effect due to whatever I use as my defenses, which relates back to doing it all as an objective observer [a researcher].

THER.: What you are saying is this is similar to the death of a loved one — the kind of experience that is sort of cleansing, like that of a woman when her husband dies who can cry very freely, very openly. Experiencing the depression is associated with the loss of a loved one. After that she is O.K. as opposed to the kind of a stalwart that holds it back, doesn't let it show, often the case with husbands whose wives die, because they can't cry openly, it is not their appropriate role to do so.

Moss: I think I belong in the former category rather than the latter. I think I respond with a full range of emotion regardless of what the situation may be. But I have learned over the years to hold it in, not to give other people the impression that I do feel strongly about things. I think that I fall into the category of the woman that you were referring to, rather than a man.

THER.: Well now, that doesn't jibe with this where you said that you really haven't experienced the depression of — that is, a loss of the higher functions. It is sort of the death of your superior skills, whereas initially you thought there would be some recovery, so there really wasn't a death, it was just sort of a temporary illness. Now you are saying that it is a permanent loss, at least it will never be the same again.

Moss: I'll have to think about that for a while. I'm not sure whether it is really a loss or not. In a sense I have always maintained in my fantasy that I would recover. And the way we are relating now, I think there is very little in my manner that would indicate any sort of a loss. Right?

THER.: That's right.

Moss: But for whatever reason, the fear that I will show a loss comes forward and intervenes in any sort of professional relationship.

Ther.: O.K. So what you are saying is that on the one hand you try to perpetuate this fantasy that you are perfectly all right, and on the other hand you still know it's a fantasy and you are still afraid that it may not be the truth.

Moss: Actually, I am not convinced that I cannot recover to a remarkable degree.

Ther.: Wait, you are not convinced that you cannot recover?

Moss: My fantasy is so strong that if you really confront me with it I'll say, "Well, maybe it isn't a fantasy at all, maybe it's reality," you see, and that what I've maintained to you up to this point is a fantasy.

Ther.: O.K. If that is the case, why are you seeing me? Why do you need me?

Moss: Because someone must be able to spell out what the reality is. If it is a fantasy, then I should give it up. You must maintain that it is a fantasy and I should reestablish contact with reality.

Ther.: What you are asking now is that what you really want me to do is help you discriminate so that you can say, "All right, I'm functioning all right here and it's realistic to say I'm just as good as I always was in this particular situation, but in other situations I'm not," whatever those situations are, and you want me to help you discriminate between them. "Don't try to kid yourself, Scott Moss, you've got a deficit here, you always will, that's the way life is, let's live with it."

Moss: What is the form of the deficit and is the deficit physiological or organic or is it functional? I'm sorry to pop all of this onto you during our discussion and yet these things have preoccupied me from the beginning.

Ther.: I'm just trying to put the pieces together here. We were initially sort of concluding that it was a good deal functional and apparently a good number of the doctors you have seen in the past — what one fantasy is that it is a good deal functional, in fact, that is, kind of the fantasy on which we based the initial part of this therapy, was that it was functional and it is something that is associated with anxiety. If we eliminate the anxiety and it was functional, it will go away. Now we are questioning the initial fantasy — is it functional? And it also sounds to me as though sometimes you really believe this fantasy but you do get into relationships where you do block or things are difficult and you begin to question the fantasy — is it really functional?

Moss: It seems to me that in relating to others that sooner or later I block and at that juncture it seems to me there is no alternative and I am reduced to despair for the moment, and I conclude that it is all organic.

Ther.:   Why would you conclude that? Why do you reach that conclusion rather than "It is functional and I must work harder?"

Moss: Only in contrast to my former self. I never experienced things like I experience now and the only thing that intervened was the stroke.

Ther.:   In other words, "I can't believe it is my incapabilities; therefore, it must be something physiological." And that sort of relieves you from the responsibility of your behavior.

Moss: But if I really believed it was organic, physiological, then it makes no sense to me that I haven't become depressed.

Ther.:   All right, good. So it sounds like your fantasy that it is functional is your strongest defense mechanism against the depression. As long as you can hold onto it you are protected from ever falling into the moroseness of "My God, I'll never be a whole man again!"

Moss: I never looked at it quite like that before, but it may have a lot of merit to it.

Ther.:   So what in a sense we're saying is, there may be anxiety basically with the loss of the maintenance of the fantasy, and so by saying that you need to talk about the accident as if the fantasy about it being functional were not there — you need to talk about the accident as an organic experience that is not recoverable.

Moss: That's a possibility but I would say the need to talk about the accident is in order to relieve the anxiety and to prove that it was all functional, that I don't really suffer much in terms of organic deficiency.

Ther.:   I see, you want to talk about it so that you can strengthen your fantasy.

Moss: Or is it a fantasy. I don't know.

Ther.: O.K. So you can make the fantasy become reality, so you can believe it as though it is really real.

Moss: What I am saying is that to continue doing as I have done over the past two and a half years is really untenable and what I want to do is to prove that I have only a very negligible deficit, and what is a fantasy may prove to be the reality.

Ther.: That puts us in a different ball park.

Moss: Yes, but it puts us much closer to the valid problem. The very fact that we can discuss this at length and in some depth would be some evidence that I haven't suffered nearly the degree of loss which I maintain every day in my contact with other colleagues or even students.

Ther.: Exactly! What it also means is that by constantly proving to yourself that you're able to talk and to function, the longer you can do this the more the fantasy becomes reality. You can't help but see the data that you are talking and are functioning, and the more you do this the more it must be reality.

Moss: I am able to do this with you because of the rapport which has increased to such an extent that I can let down and be myself, and for whatever reason the threat that is posed by other professional people doesn't allow me to —

Ther.: The threat to the fantasy!

Moss: I'm not sure of that.

Ther.: In other words, the threat of their finding out that you really can't carry on a conversation with them. You said earlier that you are always putting up a front, always putting on a show, and what if they found out that you blocked; the extensive notes that you prepare so that you'll look good to be able to answer all of the questions right, so nobody will know. In a sense it sounds like a threat to the fantasy.

Moss: I'm not quite sure that is correct, at least I'm not sure as to how you are using "fantasy."

Ther.: It's a threat to your belief that you can function normally.

Moss: I really don't expect either you or I to be able to formulate exactly what is going on at the moment. We'll both have to think about it in the interim. You mean the notes that I've prepared ahead of time [class notes, telephone conversations, notes preparatory to talking to some faculty member], all to prevent me from blocking.

THER.: That's what I have been talking about precisely.

Moss: I frequently make up such notes but very often don't use them, at least not publicly. They would perceive that I couldn't keep myself organized and I must write it all down ahead of time. It means that I have a demonstrable deficiency.

THER.: And the very thing that you are working very hard to maintain to Scott Moss is that you don't have a deficiency. You've got a belief that you really want to be real, but you're not really sure that that belief is real. It's kind of like a little egg shell, and you don't want it to be cracked, so you go about building elaborate defenses, like copious notes, to protect that little egg shell. It's a belief that you don't want contradicted, and you're doing all of this to keep the belief from being contradicted. We need to expose the belief, the opportunity to be tested. As long as you don't allow it to be tested, it will never be anything that you can become sure of.

Moss: Now and then I do attempt to test the belief. I occasionally arrive at a meeting without any prepared notes and sometimes it goes appropriately but at other times I block, and when I block everything comes apart. So I am forced back into extensive preparation for the next time.

THER.: Now I think we are really getting somewhere. What it says to me is, what does the belief mean? This takes us back to talking about the implications of the accident, so let's look at the importance of the belief. But also let's look at ways that we can give your belief more and more critical tests and to allow it to become a stronger belief, because it has passed stronger tests. Let's push it to its limits, and then we can start to discriminate where the limits are. Perhaps before the accident your limits were way out, practically unlimited, and now the limits aren't that far but how far are they? We're going to have to test the limits and that means that you'll have to go out and place yourself in uncomfortable positions.

Moss: I feel much better about this hour than I did about any of the previous hours.

THER.: You're right, the perspective is much better. Also, as you see it it is a matter of rapport, your ability to talk about such things.

I can't ever imagine thinking of you as an aphasic based on our just now conversation, except for the content. In terms of your style and manner and performance, it is practically impossible to see you as an aphasic.

III

At the eighth session I presented the therapist with a series of ratings which I had made of my professional contacts throughout the intervening week. The ratings, shown in Table 2, were done on a rough scale of 1 through 7, with 1 being "very anxious" or the performance was "miserable" through 7 when the judgment of the performance was "excellent" or "very satisfied" (no anxiety). The therapist was quite delighted by my attempt at behavioral evaluation and expressed amazement at the consistent high level of the appraisals. I, too, was filled with wonder, especially since I had deliberately attempted the ratings from the viewpoint of a professional person rather than from the criteria of a client's (aphasic's) point of view, which I had been emphasizing the week before. So this gave rise again to the question of what the source of my anxiety was and what was keeping it going.

TABLE 2. RATINGS ON A 7-POINT SCALE AS TO HOW
I FELT ABOUT MY PERFORMANCE IN PROFESSIONAL CONTACTS

(1 = VERY ANXIOUS; 7 = VERY SATISFIED)

Monday, April 20 (1970):		*Ratings*
6:30- 8:15	Prepared for my lecture on community mental health. I didn't quite complete it.	5
9:00-10:00	Met with Dick Block on his review of the book *Episode* (the autobiographical account of a stroke).	6
10:00-11:00	Listened to a tape of B.G. interacting with his clients Relaxation!	7
11:00-11:30	Supervised B.G. in his conduct of psychotherapy (no prepared discussion).	7
11:30-12:00	Supervised D.R. about his two clients (again no prepared notes).	6
12:00- 1:00	Final preparation for the lecture. Also saw a staff member from the nearby state mental health center and a student who wanted to borrow some material on sleep and dreams.	6

1:00- 3:00	Delivered the lecture on community mental health (I felt free to deviate somewhat from the text). Relaxation!	5
3:00- 4:45	Met with the American Psychological Association site visitors on their annual visit to assess the clinical program. Two of them were old acquaintances. Handled it adequately but again felt the need to apologize for my stroke.	5
6:30- 9:00	Listened to Susan's tape on her interviews.	5

Tuesday, April 21:

9:00-10:00	Met with the students who are affiliated with the Francis Nelson Health Center (a crisis-intervention center); Julian, the co-sponsor of the group, was tied up with the site visitors, leaving the direction on my shoulders.	4
10:00-11:00	Continued listening to Susan's tape. I deliberately did not write anything down.	5
	I also saw another staff member. He lent me a book which contained a chapter on the behavioral treatment of aphasia. He (again) stated that behaviorally I gave little evidence of my stroke.	6
11:00-11:30	Met with Susan. In contrast with previous session, I felt elated about this one.	7
12:00- 1:00	Corrected written diagnostic summaries prepared by two students.	6
1:00- 1:30	Met with Julian and told him of my leaving. He again maintained that my stroke provided me with a convenient rationalization. He (again) placed most of my difficulty on the ideological difference in this department.	7
1:30- 2:00	Read the student's reports on previous sessions with her client preparatory to seeing her. It is a most difficult case. Relaxation!	5
2:00- 2:45	The student didn't appear — she was tied up with seeing her case. I finally decided to go home.	
3:45- 5:15	Listened to the tape of my own psychotherapy.	6
6:45- 8:00	Began reading J.A.'s dissertation (found it was extremely difficult to follow).	5

TABLE 2. (continued)

Wednesday, April 22:

9:00- 2:30   Stayed at home and spent the entire day reading
and rereading J.A.'s dissertation. The thesis is
difficult. It is complex and his handling is
compulsive, but little by little it began to make
sense.   5

(I then goofed off (giving myself some reinforcement?)
and took in Joel's track meet. He again won three
first places. Hurrah! I did this in place of attending
the clinical staff meeting — my first absence
since my recovery from my stroke.)   (7)

7:00- 9:30   Conducted the seminar on hypnosymbolism. I
again succeeded in deviating from my notes a bit.   6

Thursday, April 23:

6:00- 7:00   Continued worry about J.A. dissertation and
devoted one more hour to going over it.   5

8:00-10:00   J.A. dissertation committee meeting. One of the
staff members was absent (I wish I could make it
two). But the meeting went exceptionally well,
including what I had to contribute to it.   6

Relaxation!

10:30-11:00 Met with J.D. on her case. I again did not prepare
notes. She is a real pleasure.   5

11:00-11:45 (B.O. again absented himself from supervision. I
eventually learned that he didn't hold a session last
week. I am as frustrated at him as I am pleased
by the previous student.)

(I went home and worked on the yard. I planted in
the garden.)

3:00- 5:00   Attended the psycholinguistic seminar on aphasia.
Found it was complex and also that I had very
little relevant background.   4

6:30- 9:00   Listened to two tapes: one for the forthcoming
meeting with John Levy (the second student who is
reviewing articles on aphasia), and Bill Brewer
talking about language and thought.   6

Friday, April 24:

6:45- 7:00   Up earlier to prepare Julie's problems in division.

7:30- 9:00	Continued listening to John Levy's tape of the last session and preparing for the session with him next hour.	6
10:00-11:30	Met with John in discussion of his current book, *Stroke.* Later set up a tape for him to listen to.	5
11:30-12:30	Received the galley of my forthcoming book, *Dreams, Images, and Fantasy.* Went through it peripherally.	6
12:30- 1:45	Listened to the tape of a client whom I am seeing for weight reduction through hypnosis. Relaxation!	7
2:00- 2:30	(The client didn't show up. I found myself wondering: Was it due to the "dynamics" or was it related somehow to my accident?)	
3:00- 6:00	(Spent the remainder of the afternoon painting and fixing the house.)	
8:00- 9:30	Began reading the galleys with my wife. What a dead and dull business.	4

Saturday, April 25:

5:00- 6:15	The rain woke me up. I went downstairs and read the galleys until the rain let up.	4
10:00	This therapy session.	4

Session 8, April 24, 1970

THER.: You asked the question about where we go. I'd like to do a combination of getting you to the point of differential relaxation. In other words, relaxation by recall. So you'd only have to take fifteen minutes to relax yourself. And the other thing would be for you to sit down and read parts of Ellis's *Guide to Rational Living.* It's paperback, and we'll focus on the irrational ideas that he talks about, of labeling situations as bad or as your performance in situations as bad, and the consequences.

Moss: All right. I'll be glad to look it over. I haven't looked at it for a long, long time.

THER.: You'll recall a lot of it, but I think I'd like us to talk about it. I think it would be applicable because a few weeks ago if you'd told me you rated your performances on a 1 to 7 scale, I would think there would be many more 1's.

Moss: And this surprised me, too; I had the same reaction. This is very similar, I think, to the fact that I was initially very hesitant about talking with people, and then for Christmas a year ago my wife purchased a tape recorder concealed in a valise, did I tell you?

THER.: No, I didn't know that.

MOSS: Yes, and so I lugged this around with me almost everywhere I went and recorded, unbeknownst to the other parties, samples of our discussion, and then I'd go home and listen to them. And I was amazed that I really sounded adequate, quite adequate as a matter of fact. And I did this in relation to meetings with Julian, meetings with Don, meetings with Mort, staff meetings, other sorts of meetings, and I was really amazed that I came through as clearly as I did. This still left me filled with the anxiety. Why was I still anxious? Originally I had thought before I did this that the reason I was anxious was because I simply was — I'm trying to find the right words — halting in my speech, that my speech was mixed up, I often blocked, etc.

THER.: Yes, you did mention this.

MOSS: But when I listened to myself on tape, and I've kept a good many of them on file, it was really very difficult for me to detect how I sounded a year or year and a half ago versus how I sound now. They all sound fairly adequate. And being confronted with this data, this caused me to sit down and think again — what's the source of my anxiety? And what I finally came around to was that it wasn't the fact that I was really blocking and halting the way I thought I was, but that it was the constant searching for words, something that wasn't really reflected in my speech, which causes me to feel anxious. Each word that I say — it's very difficult to predict that I'll know what will come after it or that I might not block in the immediate future. And I think this was the cause, as far as I could determine, of my anxiety.

THER.: Your computer is working overtime and your connections you're not real sure about.

MOSS: Right.

THER.: You know, you may have a good point. There are three things: (*a*) you are having to work harder to talk, (*b*) you're not sure about whether or not the right thing will come out, and (*c*) when you do slip, when you do block, then it's a catastrophe which

you remember, rather than the other fifteen minutes of good conversation, and then that reinforces your questioning about whether
your connections are good.

Moss: Yes, I think this is very, very appropriate, what you're
saying now. I think this may be largely the basis for the anxiety
that I feel.

THER.: Right, you get reinforced for worrying — you block just often
enough to keep yourself concerned about it.

Moss: Yes.

THER.: You know, I think you have a point here, that maybe you
ought to keep on using your valise with the hidden recorder and give
yourself feedback.

Moss: I've listened to myself again and again in many situations
and I'm convinced I don't block nearly as much as I maintain.
Yet, just listening to myself not blocking, doesn't do away with
the anxiety. I'm still really concerned that I may not block now,
but I may block in the immediate future. This tells me that I can
go for long periods of time and perform fairly well — very well.

THER.: You could go for a month and then maybe the next week —

Moss: Yes, I think the situation is at this juncture: I can talk
reasonably well with individuals, but talking in front of groups or
crowds and having to talk spontaneously is the basis for much of
my anxiety.

THER.: O.K. So it's the blocking in front of the crowd, the lecture
or the speech.

Moss: Yes, but remember, as long as I have time to prepare what
I am going to say, I'm all right. But it's the spontaneousness of it in
front of a group that causes me to block.

THER.: In a sense the decision to go back to California would put
you in less frequent situations of having to perhaps respond spontaneously to groups.

Moss: Yes, and perhaps there's another quality. I think that in the
prison system I'll be relating largely to people who are less trained
academically than here.

THER.: I don't buy that as a valid reason. That's a reason which you
created because you're making the assumption that you can't really
communicate adequately or comfortably to people around here

who are "intellectually bright." In other words you are saying, "I'm not as good so therefore I'm leaving." I'm saying that the situations occur more frequently around here — that you speak to a group spontaneously more than out in California. I mean it's the situation that disturbs you, not the fact that you're less capable.

In other words, if you've got a person who's afraid of snakes, you don't have him living in the Okefenokee swamps. It doesn't mean he's any less of a person, it just means that you let him live someplace where he doesn't have to live around snakes. You see what I'm saying?

Moss: I'm not quite sure.

Ther.: You're saying that "if I go out to California where I'm dealing with people who are not as sharp as people in Illinois, I'm going to be better off because I'm not quite as sharp as I used to be."

Moss: Yes, I believe that.

Ther.: You believe that and I'm saying that's not quite valid. There are situations which make you more anxious now than they used to, but that doesn't mean that you're any less sharp. Because we've talked about this before and we've concluded that there's a good deal of (*a*) avoidance of the opportunity to be stuck in a spontaneous situation where you have to respond in front of a group spontaneously, and (*b*) we've just looked at this to see that most of the time in spontaneous group situations you function all right.

Moss: And that's probably true, and yet if we took a hypothetical group and I was supposed to respond spontaneously, at the end of the dialogue I would think that probably my responses were far from adequate.

Ther.: Probably.

Moss: Now if I listened to a tape of what I said, I would be amazed that I responded as well as I did, but then I would take the attitude that I did all right in this instance but in the next instance —

Ther.: That's exactly right. Now see the point is that you're not allowing yourself many instances to begin with, because you try to be prepared and you try to avoid getting involved in those situations.

Moss: That's right.

Ther.: O.K. So you've actually avoided the shock because you're prepared, and even when you do get into the situation where you are not prepared and there is the possibility of getting shocked, if you don't get shocked that time, you're almost sure you will the next time. And it means that as the learning theorists point out, you're going to have to go through many, many trials of not getting shocked in a situation before you begin to become a believer that "maybe I won't get shocked." Because you've gone through the last thirty times and haven't gotten shocked.

Moss : And if I get shocked the thirty-first time, I'll write it off to the fact that I have gone through the preceding thirty situations, which would be much the way it was originally before the accident.

Ther. : But the one thing is that you really keep yourself from getting into these situations by being very careful and planning and avoiding the possibility of a shock. Therefore, you never really find out if you will get shocked.

Moss : Yes. For example, the other day I had a telephone call from a girl who was associated with 101 or 103, or whatever is an introductory psych. course, and she was looking for a speaker on dreams. She wanted to know if I would come and talk to a group. For a moment I was tempted and then I remembered everything else I had to do and I said, "Well, I really can't do it." I suggested perhaps Julian or Doug or somebody else might respond to her call. And the reason I didn't do it was first, I would be thrust into a situation where I'd have to confront a group, and second of all, if I did this, then I would have to sit down and spend long hours of preparation before I went out and met the group.

Ther. : Let me go back to my initial point, though. The point I am making is that it's not that you're a less capable person, not that you're sort of a second-class rather than a first-class intellect. I'm saying that it's not that — that's not the reason you're going to California, I hope not.

Moss : I'm sure it entered into it.

Ther. : Well, you told me a minute ago that this is the reason you gave. And I'm saying that's the kind of self-label, of self-stimulation, that is going to convince you that you're always going to be a second-class citizen. That you're never going to be as you used to be. These are the kinds of things that you're saying to yourself. "I'm not as good as I used to be. I'm no longer what I was." You see what I'm saying?

MOSS: Let me give two qualifications to what you're saying, if I can.

THER.: All right.

MOSS: First of all, I may be as intellectually bright as I was before. I think, over a period of time, I have returned more or less to my former intellectual ability. But where I am not as capable as I was before is in expressing my thoughts to other people in a way which is convincing. The second reason is that it's a peculiarity which is inherent in this situation and not in the majority of situations.

It's simply the fact that I adhere to a different theoretical position.

THER.: Oh, yes, that was here before you ever got here.

MOSS: And it's simply the fact that I found the faculty and students were of quite a different orientation. So anything that I had to say, I would be confronted. There was no source of reinforcement in this situation for me.

THER.: In fact a lot of demands were put on you to justify your position.

MOSS: That's right, do you see, and —

THER.: O.K. I got you. In other words, your skills of argumentation and confrontation and persuasion of another person may not be as sharp now as they used to be. Intellectually it's all there, it's just the rapid argument, the coming up with new reasons and new explanations constantly gets to you. O.K., that I might buy. But it's not because you're somewhat half a man.

MOSS: I would agree with you theoretically, but I think these two qualifications are very important in my level of present functioning, and if, for example, this accident had occurred in a different situation, for example, while I was still with NIMH, I think I would have found a much more comfortable and reinforcing situation than I happened to be in at the time this all happened.

THER.: Yes, you're in enemy territory here and this is no place to have an accident. That's a way of looking at it, well, I don't mean enemy territory but I mean at least a different orientation.

MOSS: Well, enemy territory expresses it at a gut reaction level rather than an intellectual level.

THER.: O.K. I still want to try to get you to focus on the positive, to relabel your performance, and to relabel the expectations of other people. And along with it to combine the differential relaxation and the relaxation by recall. I think that the relaxation is an important component and a comfortable component. Something that has concerned me with regard to your labeling yourself and your state of being, has been these articles you've been reading on aphasia. Particularly the one that you said was most descriptive of your situation about the young Navy guy who got hurt on a motorcycle or something (p. 190). The reason why it's concerned me is his resulting brain damage and problems; there's no way of telling from the article the extent of brain damage. He had a lot of problems, focused a good deal on the negative and a good deal on the fact that they gave him an I.Q. test after the accident and he considered his intelligence to be around 100 or a little bit below. This was a significant drop from the way he had been before the accident. And what you just said a little while ago is that you feel you are about as intelligent now as you were before the accident.

Moss: I feel I'm somewhat slower in grasping the points that are made.

Ther.: I'm concerned, though, about this constant focus.

Moss: And so you think this is aversive or nonreinforcing?

Ther.: Well, it's reinforcing of the negative attitude.

Moss: Yes, I read these articles and always in the back of my mind is an attempt to identify what sort of symptoms does he have which are parallel to my own.

Ther.: It's a kind of intellectual rumination, probably at a productive level, because you'll probably write something about it. But I'm concerned about it; I get the feeling that rather than focusing on how life is the way it used to be, you're focusing on how life isn't the way it used to be because now you're an aphasic. "I'm not Scott Moss, I'm now aphasic Scott Moss."

Moss: I'm an aphasic *case,* which even eliminates the human level.

Ther.: I don't like it if we're going to focus on how Scott Moss is a whole functioning individual who has had his appendix removed or something like this. He is no longer an appendicitis *case,* he's — you're Scott Moss.

Moss: I think the result of having a stroke is somewhat different

from being an appendix case. It's even different if I had an arm
or leg removed, because something that's happened to your brain
in a sense is getting at you, yourself, what you are. You can adjust
to the loss of an eye, an arm or leg. But it's much more difficult,
I think, for a trauma or a lesion which affects your brain, because
the brain is, in a sense, your whole personality, *who you are*.

THER.: Well, O.K. I kind of see things in terms of who you see
yourself as, an educator, a learned man, the brain is more important. I suspect that for the guy who earns his bread by shoveling coal
or laying bricks, the loss of an arm would be equally disastrous. So
actually, this hit you where it hurt the most. You can write with
one hand, and you can dictate letters, so if you'd lost an arm
you'd still be O.K.

Moss: Yes, in a sense, it would have been much more — what's the
word now — I would have adjusted much better if I had lost an
arm or leg instead of my intellect. And at this time I don't think
my intellect is really impaired as much as my ability to communicate.

THER.: Communication is your bag.

Moss: It is for everyone, here.

THER.: That's right, and so any analogy pales in comparison.

Moss: But you are correct that the bricklayer would be disadvantaged by the loss of an arm. And that is, I think, a good comparison to me.

THER.: But it still concerns me about the focus on this, particularly
since we said several times that you feel to a fairly large extent that
you've recovered a great deal of your original facility. Not totally,
you're still slower. Where do we draw the line? Where do we stop
focusing on the slowness and focus on the fact that you can think
and that you can communicate somewhat?

Moss: And this is a large part of why we entered therapy together,
I think — my trying to define what physiological residuals I still
have and how much is due to anxiety.

THER.: From the looks of this sort of thing there is probably a
10 percent residual and that's the 10 percent when you block. I
think in the last forty minutes you've blocked twice, in two statements. Verbally, I mean behaviorally. Now I don't know how many
times you've blocked cognitively, but behaviorally I've heard you

block twice. You said this is why we got together, to figure out what was residual and what was anxiety, and I'm saying it sounds as though there is some anxiety there that is an influence, but I think we've gotten some effect from relaxation. You know, I want us to continue this. Given situations, let's say, when you're totally relaxed and in a conversation, I would say you might suspect maybe 5 percent of the time your accident is influencing you. That gives us 95 percent of the time that you're functioning on all eight cylinders.

Moss: What you're doing now I think is important because this, of course, is my own judgment that enters into each of these.

Ther.: That's what's important, though, because you're your hardest judge. You're your harshest critic.

Moss: Yes, I would agree. And yet I think your entering in and saying what you did, that in the last forty minutes you perceived I blocked twice, gives me some support for the fact that I should look at this more positively rather than as I did negatively. It's almost as if, coming back to this again, it is as if you or someone else listened to each of these and sat down and had your own rating. I guess I suspect that you as an outside observer would rate me lower than I rate myself, and if you didn't, well, then I would think you were just responding as a reinforcement, as a therapist. There is a different sort of judgment which enters into therapy as opposed to a professional point of view. No matter what you did, I would write it off.

Ther.: If we can get us some very unbiased observers and say tape three or four days or a week or a month and pull out random five-minute segments so we get random distribution of all these points, for one thing the frequency of your blocking is fairly low compared to the amount. So taking random segments because you couldn't expect them to listen to all of it, have them unbiasedly rate the frequency of blocking or some sort of absolute scale of 1 to 7 on performance, probably that might convince you from the point of an objective observer. I'm not sure it would convince you beyond that. I mean, I think you would still say, "Well, they didn't hear enough." I'm not really sure that would be all it would take, that's what I'm saying. It's not really until you convince yourself, find some way to convince yourself that it's really going to make any difference.

Moss: I would agree and yet I don't know at this juncture how I can convince myself, because in effect, I think, I've been trying to convince myself for two and a half years.

Ther.: In a way, yes, but while on the one hand you have been trying to convince yourself, on the other hand you continue to focus on negative things, how your symptoms are somebody else's symptoms.

Moss: It's almost a dual personality, you know — part of me is striving for normality and part of me is striving to remain an aphasic.

Ther.: Why do you think that would be? Why would you like to label yourself as an aphasic?

Moss: Why? Why?

Ther.: What does it get you?

Moss: It gets me out of a lot of situations which would be taxing, anxiety-stimulating. And it allows me to, in effect, over a couple of years, structure my situation so that I can do exactly what I want to do and to refuse, refrain from doing other things that might be anxiety-arousing.

Ther.: And some of these may have been anxiety-arousing even before the accident?

Moss: Of course.

Ther.: So it's kind of "I'm sick, don't bother me."

Moss: It was never put that blatantly, but I'm aware that I have convinced everyone now that I can't do certain things and so they don't even call on me to do these things any longer. On the other hand, realizing that this has been the effect of my behavior, then why am I not satisfied to accept what my accident has made of the situation and settle down and not exploit the situation for all its worth?

Ther.: Really get lazy?

Moss: Not lazy, because as I have told you I work just about as hard now as I did earlier, from six o'clock in the morning until eight or nine.

Ther.: "Lazy" isn't the word, I should say avoiding certain situations.

Moss: Yes, but at this juncture — let me back up a little bit — next year if I stayed here, Mort and Don had both said that I would no longer have to teach courses in community psychology and I was free to just teach the course on hypnosymbolism, which I like to do, and teach a course in abnormal psychology. You see this in a sense would be excellent. It would allow me to do with all the other time exactly what I wanted to do: write books, engage in research, and so on, and yet for whatever reason, this wasn't palatable to me. I felt that I must get out of the situation and get into a more difficult situation, but one that I could handle more adroitly or better than what I had worked myself into by remaining here. This is the other side of it.

THER.: I'm wondering if there were — there are two things. You still see yourself as a person who is very conscientious and who will go out and work very hard to get what he wants, and isn't one to push aside something simply because it isn't the most pleasant thing in the world. It's kind of a Protestant ethic of "Work hard, do even unpleasant things, and the rewards will come." And yet that is an unpleasant ethic. What I'm saying is that on the one hand you have a value which reinforces you for doing the dirty work and on the other hand the unpleasantness of the work itself which makes you want to avoid it.

It's kind of an approach-avoidance situation; you know that you ought to do it, but you really don't want to. So not to do it makes you feel a little guilty and a little bad, because you're not really meeting that value which you hold so high. Therefore, not to teach the course that you don't want to teach anyway and to have a very pleasant situation like teaching Abnormal and having all this time to yourself really isn't such a pleasant thing, because you're not reaching your value. It makes you something less than a whole person. To not teach a course because you're aphasic isn't a very pleasant reason. So in a way it becomes a way of getting out of unpleasant situations, but on the other hand it isn't a very good reason.

Moss: Or at least not acceptable in the way that you are phrasing it.

THER.: Yes, it is not acceptable.

Moss: I don't know whether it is true or part of it is true; I'll have to think it over.

THER. I don't know — I'm just trying to create a hypothesis, and looking upon it as to why you would maintain your aphasia and yet on the other hand dislike the maintenance. What does it benefit you to maintain it? And why in maintaining it does it still make you feel bad? The other thing is as long as you maintain the aphasia this value of being intellectually competent goes against that value. And that would definitely make you feel bad, because you hold that very highly.

Moss: There's a lot in what you've said but again I'm not sure what, if anything, describes my situation, and yet I'm quite willing to bet that any type of illness brings its own rewards. Whether the person admits it, he still uses his illness in various ways to define the situation in the way he wants. For example, I can't help but think back to my grandmother. My grandmother suffered a stroke and my mother took care of her for eleven years before she died. Over time, I became aware that she used her stroke to manipulate my mother more and more, and in the end it was as if one was treating an infantile woman. So from that alone it tells me that whether she recognized it or not, this was nevertheless the result.

Now in terms of my own mother, I'm aware that as the years go on, various health difficulties are intruding in her life and into our relationship. More and more, whether she recognizes it or not, she often relates in such a way as to make me feel guilty if I don't do certain things that she wishes. So again in these instances that are so very close to home, I am aware that whether the person professes or acknowledges it, he is using his illness to his own gain. It has an insidious effect on his interpersonal relationships. It is true that in a sense, unconsciously, not through my own volition, I have used my stroke and my impairment in communication to define the situation that I'm in as being the best for me. Now everyone does this all the time, but the stroke —

Ther.: Does provide a new reason. And the thing in this is the immediate consequences may be good. What I mean is that your mother is in a situation where she manipulates you and she gets what she wants — she gets enough reinforcement so she keeps it up. But she's aware that that is not how to treat her son and as a consequence feels bad later on upon reflecting on treating you this way. This is the neurotic problem, that we function to a large extent for what occurs immediately; later on our "conscience" makes us pay for it, because we know that's not the right way to act. It's kind of acting angry with somebody and saying exactly what you think, but later on you know that wasn't the way to act.

Moss: Yes, when a person suffers an illness he reacts in insidious ways to get what he wants, without really confronting other people with the reason he wants to do it a certain way, and I am not sure that he really ever tells himself.

Ther.: I think we are saying the same things. You would have liked to give that talk about dreams but the immediate thinking about all the time involved and the anxiety associated with going out to give the talk added up to a negative response. You avoided something aversive. But you know in the back of your mind was also the reason that "I, Scott Moss, am an aphasic and I just can't go out and give talks like other people can." Later on you think back and you say, "I really wanted to give that talk."

Moss: "If only it hadn't have been for my accident." At an earlier date I could have gone gladly.

Ther. Or so you think you would have.

Moss: So who's fooling whom? What is the real effect of the accident?

Ther.: And that's a difficult question. It's probably an unanswerable question. What I think you are going to have to start saying to yourself is that "If I decide that it is an aversive situation, my decision must be made not because I am an aphasic, but because I don't want to spend the time and energy doing it."

Moss: Do you mean just ignoring the fact that I suffer from the residuals of aphasia?

Ther.: I'm not calling it a residual of aphasia, unless you want to call anxiety a residual of aphasia. All I'm saying is that you feel anxious in that situation and you choose to avoid it. There is nothing wrong with your choosing to do one thing and not the other. What difference does it make whether the reason is a good one or a bad one?

Moss: It does make a difference to me. One must give a valid reason and the reason is aphasia or the residuals and not just anxiety. It is, in effect, how I really think about it and this gives me a valid reason. I don't think the fact of anxiety would be sufficient.

Ther.: The question still remains that if aphasia is the reason then you shouldn't go and chastise yourself for this reason.

Moss: But I can't get out of that.

Ther.: Why can't you?

MOSS: It comes down to the fact that I really don't accept the fact that I am aphasic.

THER.: Or if you are, it will keep you from doing other things that you to want to do.

MOSS: Yes.

THER.: And therefore, you have a choice to make: either use aphasia as the reason and feel bad as a consequence because it goes against basic values or quit using aphasia as the reason and face the fact that you feel anxiety in certain situations, that you do work hard all day and can't do everything.

MOSS: But without extended preparation, I am afraid that I will block.

THER.: So therefore don't ever put yourself in the situation where you can overcome that fear. Don't ever let yourself get out on the floor and find out that you might *not* block. Just keep on chastising yourself and basing it on a fear that you'll never find out if it is realistic or not. It means taking the risk of going out and perhaps blocking.

MOSS: I guess that I'm really afraid of blocking, rather than that I do block, that I just can't bring myself to confront that situation without thorough preparation. And I can't read off the paper what I intended to say; it wasn't sufficient for me to compose cryptic little notes because that didn't provide me the assurance that I would remember what I wanted to say. I notice the time is slipping by — again it is my feeling that the time we spent this hour is most profitable. I think again we are talking about things that are much more akin to the problem.

THER.: I think you're right. Given relaxation as a component of the whole situation, I think that we should concentrate on your perception of what you're doing and why you're doing it and how you feel about it. I want you to go ahead and reread Ellis because that's what Ellis is talking about. How to get this stuff under control. When you use the reason that you are aphasic it undermines so many things that it is not acceptable and you feel miserable, plus the factor that it underlines something that is very aversive and anxiety-provoking — that you are incapable. This is a very uncomfortable and unpleasant feeling.

MOSS: And what was the point about my reading self-reports of aphasics?

THER.: By your reading these self-reports, you are identifying yourself with a lot of negative things, that people with much more brain
damage suffer. I'd rather you'd sit and read articles about normal
people, like Albert Einstein, and identify with them. There's always
hope for the kid who flunked high school math because Albert Einstein flunked high school math. Therefore, I may be another Albert
Einstein, I may be able to function on his level. What you're doing is
reading articles about aphasics who are saying they can't do one
thing and another, and you are saying that you can't do that either,
and identifying with the symptomatic qualities of those people. And
rather than being a boosting effect, it seems to be a depressing effect.

Moss: I think you may be right — that there may be a profound element of truth in that. I'll have to think about this.

IV

I continued to accumulate ratings of all of my professional contacts on
the 7-point scale during the three remaining treatment sessions (May 9,
23, and 30). It continued to astonish both of us that almost all of the
evaluations fell in either the "neutral" or positive units; the only instance of "anxious" ratings was in connection with the weekly clinical
staff meetings. The prior aversive conditioning during the period of my
recuperation from my stroke when I was "truly aphasic" (essentially
the first six months to a year) was apparently strong enough so that
even these few negative situations were enough to sustain my great ap-
prehensiveness in interpersonal relations.

TABLE 3. ACCUMULATED ANXIETY RATINGS

	1 very anxious	2 anxious	3 somewhat anxious	4 neutral	5 somewhat satisfied	6 satisfied	7 very satisfied
total ratings	0	2	2	16	33	24	10

Bear in mind that the contacts reflected on the right-hand side of the
scale were not devoid of anxiety; there was some uneasiness in each
and every one, but not enough really to impair performance grossly.
Part of the explanation also resided in the careful way that I had man-

aged to structure and limit my professional contacts; that is, I consciously avoided any anxiety-provoking situations beyond a certain level. In my way of thinking, this was very appropriate, since it was gauged on how much upset I could handle before my performance might become disorganized. And over time, as I felt able, I was involving myself with more and more "risk" elements. But as the therapist pointed out, this was a "two-edged sword": it protected me from overwhelming anxiety but at the same time prevented me from ever testing how much I was capable of dealing with. What was the reality of my incapacity? It is true that I generalized from the staff meetings and concluded that I could not handle anything else in the way of external, formal contacts because of the expectation that I might block: however, I had already learned to refrain from preparing for my psychotherapy supervisory sessions in great detail, since I had found out that they went almost as well when I didn't have any notes to refer to.

There were two additional highlights at the ninth session. In rereading Ellis's book (1962), I found that only one of his ten "irrational" principles really struck home, although I thought his elaboration on it was largely irrelevant. The principle was this:

Give up the notion of trying to be thoroughly competent, adequate, and achieving in all possible respects. Try to *do* rather than to do *perfectly*. Try to better your own performances rather than those of others. Strive, if you will, to be a better artist, ballplayer, or business man than you now are; but do not delude yourself that you will be a better *person* if you achieve your goal. Strongly desire and work for success in your chosen fields; but be ready to accept failures as undesirable but not dreadful — as having nothing whatever to do with your intrinsic value as a human being. [p. 186]

This gave rise to speculation as to some of my personality traits in this and subsequent sessions. For example, I readily admitted that even before the accident I tended to do homework rather thoroughly. So in a sense I was "compulsive," but I looked on this as a rather rare state of excellence, since I was usually prepared for most eventualities. This in turn again reflects upon my value in always being intellectually competent, and undoubtedly I did confuse this with the worth of being a better or more esteemed person. I resolved to try in each situation simply to *do* adequately, giving up the business of trying to do *perfectly.*

In the session I also announced with some pride the acceptance of a "difficult assignment," namely, agreeing to go on a National Institute of Mental Health site visit to a research project in Los Angeles the following week. The therapist was delighted, and a good deal of time was spent in how I would deal with the situation. Three possibilities eventually presented themselves: (1) I could go and say nothing; or, if I got the gumption to speak up, then (2) I could look on myself as a summarizer or clarifier, a function which I considered as an ideal contribution to a site visit; or (3) I could take a middle-of-the-road role, being a compiler and trying to keep the conversation on task which I deemed more likely. Of course, even the contemplation gave rise to concern. We finished the session by engaging for the first time in relaxation by recall (focusing my attention on quickly relaxing the four major muscle groups without actually tensing them).

When we met two weeks later for the next to the last session, the conversation turned immediately to the outcome of the site visit. It was my subjective judgment that probably I would rate my performance as a 1 or 2, but acknowledged that other participants might not agree. The visit had concerned a complicated research project with a long history (NIMH had actually forwarded twenty-five different documents as background information). It was not a regular site visit to a project before it was funded; instead, the grant was two years old and the recipients had already received four different site visits. NIMH was deeply troubled about the project and didn't want to go on tossing good money after bad. In addition, the objectives were in a politically sensitive area. I wasn't very satisfied about my contribution, but on the other hand, it was doubtful that anyone new to the project could have offered much. I spent three hectic days of about fifteen hours each, and the visit had wearied me. It seemed I blocked and stumbled a good deal in relating to Bette about the trip.

Incidentally, we had sold our house in the interim, a fact which decreased my concerns by one. (As a Christmas gift Bette had given me a series of oil painting lessons, perhaps in the hope that some latent adolescent talent might be developed into a hobby. I went for three lessons. Then we decided to sell the house without using a realtor, and

I painted an attractive, if amateur, "For Sale" sign, and placed it on my easel on the front lawn, much to the chagrin of my wife, who was afraid that the instructor, a neighbor, would take offense. We sold the house to the third viewer and I retired from the art profession, having made a fabulous profit from my first and only picture.)

In dealing with the reading which I was doing on the self-reports of aphasics, it had become increasingly apparent to me that this was in large part a form of self-help dealing with my own accident, since I could not or would not find a psychotherapist to help me handle it. In this tenth session, I made reference to Buck (p. 197) and his finding that no amount of practicing with a speech therapist had helped him; it was only when he trained himself to stop worrying about *how* he was going to say something and keep his mind focused clearly upon the concept that he began to talk again. In effect, this is the way the normal person goes about talking — not carefully and deliberately choosing his words and sentences, but keeping his objective (the concept to be communicated) always in mind. An aphasic finds it is almost impossible to keep both things in mind at the same time, and apparently the way that I had naturally chosen (and I presume the way most aphasics go about it) was one hundred percent the wrong way. The therapist seemed to be enthusiastic about Buck's perception.

In the last two sessions we spent a fair amount of time delving into specifics about my own life-style. I had been expressing my concern about intruding into another colleague's time, which led to the fact that I had always been pretty much of a loner in my accomplishments. I looked on myself as rather humble and relatively unobtrusive; in fact, I have a depreciatory attitude toward my own professional accomplishments. I have always liked to accomplish my tasks alone (like writing an article or book) and then sit back and wait for the applause and appreciation to follow; if they didn't I'd be hurt, but would then only redouble my efforts.

When I have talked to people about professional concerns, the attention that I have always paid to the sentence structure was comparable to that given to writing a formal report. It was as if I had to compensate for some insidious inferiority, and whereas I was competent to bring it off earlier, the accident deprived me of some of my language skills. Now I shied away from the possibility of blocking, since it would reveal my supposed deficiencies. If and when I was trained to do away with the elevated expectations of other people and myself, then I was assured that the speech would rapidly improve. At least from therapy I had learned to stop apologizing for my circumstances and stop focusing attention on my errors when they did occur. The problem that we were working on was my own perception of myself; and I was caught up in the old self-fulfilling prophecy role. These discussions made up my mind not to tell any additional people in California about the stroke or the fact that I still secretly thought of myself as suffering from the remains of aphasia. In actual fact, my speech was already so greatly improved that the therapist tried to impress upon me the fact that he hadn't perceived blocking frequently enough to give rise even to the remote possibility of brain damage.

Session 11, May 30, 1970

THER.: I guess what I was responding to is the hope that with the continuing use of differential relaxation and the change in your attempting now to assert yourself a little more, that you will be less traumatized, and given the appropriate alternative behaviors when you do block, that it won't become as difficult an experience. I would like it to become something that you become irritated at —

Moss: As a normal person would. And what you're saying means becoming a normal person again.

THER.: A normal person is your perspective, that's the reality that we're working with.

Moss: I'm not quite sure about what *my* perspective is.

THER.: In other words, the doctors can examine you, your students will listen to you, your peers can talk to you, and they'll all label you as a normal person. The one person who doesn't label you as normal is *you*.

Moss: I think that is probably correct.

THER.: And I'm saying the reality that we're working with is your own perception of yourself, not anybody else's.

Moss: But how does a person's perception of himself get so distorted? It amazes me, if I accept what you are saying and I think I do, then it amazes me that what happened two and a half years ago still bothers me enough —

THER.: I think we talked about this earlier. Originally there was a realistic problem, you had a lot of problems and as a consequence you developed a set of avoidance behaviors, to avoid the anxiety-producing situations. Avoidance behaviors do not go away, so by avoiding situations you never learned to cope with them.

Moss: In effect it's a phobia?

THER.: Yes, it's a phobia, a mild one but very complex in that it varies across interpersonal relationships. So that's why I'm very excited when I hear you say that you have quit making extensive notes because you have just given up on avoidance behavior and have discovered that you don't need those notes to function very well. That's why I want you to keep on constantly getting into situations with an alternate behavior — to get your feet wet, but not all the way up to your neck, just enough to experience it and discover that you can survive, and find things don't come out so badly after all.

Moss: Yes, I understand what you are saying. Somehow or other my measure of excellence enters into this and I understand that the standards that I hold for myself are far and away above what I should actually hold for myself. And yet I don't know the solution to that problem, how I can ever downgrade my performance and still be happy or satisfied with it.

THER. No, I think this will take care of itself. What would be important for it is how to enter situations and be glad that you've moved from point A to point B. You haven't reached your ultimate point but at least you've made movement.

Moss: In a sense what you are saying goes back to what I was saying last time, in terms of the ultimate goal, I never reach there. For example, writing the recent book, I just consider it as one more step in trying to prove myself to me and, professionally, to my colleagues, and when I have done a particular assignment I dismiss it from my mind because there are a thousand and one other objectives that confront me. I don't know whether that makes sense or not?

THER.: Yes, it is as you say, that you never reach your goal — it's always beyond wherever you are going. I guess what I'm saying is that you move from step A to step B, and focus on the satisfaction of having moved in that direction, rather than the dissatisfaction of not having reached your goal. Be happy for small things, be happy for what you've done, not dissatisfied for what you've not done.

Moss: And what I guess I am saying is that I did this all along. I never really achieved the ultimate goal. So wherever I am now, suffering whatever residuals of aphasia that I may have, I still strive toward achieving the ultimate goal, but I'm not *dis*satisfied. I have to pause — what I'm saying is — originally, before the stroke, I wasn't dissatisfied because I always knew that week by week I was progressing. I might never reach anything but I was satisfied knowing that I was accomplishing things. Since the stroke, the whole thing is thrown into — disconfabulation — something like that — and what has been missing for the last two and a half years is the sense of accomplishing or progressing toward anything.

Ther.: In other words, you've had to stop and make a few repairs and you haven't been able to focus on what you've wanted to do — to move on and go on to bigger and better things.

Moss: And yet if you ask me what the "bigger and better things" are, I can't answer — any more than I could three years ago.

Ther.: Well, your book is now a bigger and better thing.

Moss: At least it is a side of my experiences that I had to share and expose to the critical review of other professional people. But now that I'm done with it, I'm through with it.

Ther.: It's just another hurdle. But for two and a half years you weren't going over any hurdles and that was what was frustrating. As I say, a lot of it goes back to getting so caught up in a lack of movement or in what you were not doing that you lose perspective on what you are doing. It's like getting caught up in not being able to talk and focusing on that, and as a consequence not being able to talk, rather than trying to figure out how to go on and do things and focus on accomplishment.

Moss: I feel that what you're saying is correct. I think it could be put somewhat better, more at home with what I feel, and I'm not reproaching you, because if I could formulate it better I would do it for you now. But what you are saying is meaningful and almost correct.

Ther.: Still, to do it is a difficult problem.

Moss: Yes, and the point is that I have been working assiduously for two and a half years to accomplish this goal without much in terms of professional guidance, so I appreciate again that you're coming in and reviewing things with me and adding things that I really didn't appreciate before. It is amazing to me that it took so long to find anybody in a professional category to sit down and do this.

Ther.: That's the way things are —

Moss: But they shouldn't be, really. You and I and our colleagues are working toward meeting the needs of clients and patients, and for someone who had a very definite need for two and a half years, it is astonishing that I floundered about and couldn't find a person who would discuss things with me as you have done.

Ther.: It has a lot of implications for community psychology and the opportunity for individuals to be willing to sit and listen whether they are professionals or not. There is a need for a place where persons can go and talk about their problems. There is a vacuum of places for people to sit down and talk to people and receive good, solid reflections. And it's a shame. On the other side, there is an awful lot of reluctance to do this by persons who need to talk to someone, simply because there is still a good deal of trepidation about how they will be received. People don't ordinarily talk to people about their problems.

Moss: This is always true, and yet in terms of my own case, I think I actively sought out professional people, and yet I found them few and far between.

Ther.: That's the other side; I think there is an equal amount of trepidation for those who are called upon to sit and listen. It's a threat to them, too, because it is threatening for one person to sit and listen to another. It is much safer to sit behind the desk where you're the doctor and they're the patients. One of the problems with you was it is a little more difficult when one doctor talks to another doctor, because the placebo and role delineations are blurred. It requires more involvement of the therapist.

Moss: Do you, Jim, feel that the time we spent together was worth your while? That it has been a meaningful relationship to you?

Ther.: Oh, yes. Let me put it this way: what happens around here is that the obvious reinforcers — money, publications, teaching — are visible, and to take a client and simply have a good relationship and experience the pleasantness of talking is not as obvious or as tangible. It's not something that the academic community values. So when you asked me whether my time spent with you was experienced as valuable on the academic market, it isn't, but as an individual it is very valuable. Something that makes these other things very empty, and hollow and meaningless. That's what life is all about — warm, interpersonal relationships. That's the way that I'd look on any experience with any client up to this point. And yet the realities of the market place don't allow me to enjoy it as much as I would like to.

Moss: It sort of troubled me that in the beginning we did engage in obvious behavior techniques and little by little we have gone through these and in the last half of our sessions it has become much more a conventional therapeutic relationship. While I recognize that behavioral theory is in back of what you are doing, I would say that what you are doing is pretty much what I would do in relating to a client or a fellow being in trouble. It was a bit of a concern to me whether you felt that you were still being effective in what you were doing, not emphasizing quite as much these formal behavior modification techniques.

Ther.:   My only criterion for effectiveness is whether the client is happier. I don't care what I use or how I do it or what happens, if the person with whom I'm talking is enjoying life more, is feeling better about himself, is much more satisfied about what he is doing. It's a very simplistic view and probably oversimplified, but it is my basic precept for my doing therapy.

V

Calhoun: When Scott approached me about helping him with his problem, I was not at all sure what the best approach would be. Early, as we discussed his problem, it sounded as if there was a very complex combination of realistic anxiety due to the aphasia, conditioned anxiety aggravated by the stroke, and misperception due to labeling his behavior. At first it seemed it would be best to go right on and try systematic desensitization to see if it would work. If it were not effective, then we would decide what to do at that time.

There were other factors behind the choice of systematic desensitization in addition to its direct application in relieving Scott's anxiety. It was chosen in order to create confidence in the therapist and added rapport between them. That is, Scott had heard a lot about the technique and was possibly impressed by it, and my knowledge of the technique was one of the reasons Scott asked me to work with him. A second reason for the choice of systematic desensitization was that it provided the opportunity to train Scott in labeling and discriminating situations so that we could both assess them and communicate about them. It would also provide Scott with a new orientation toward his behaviors. The third reason for beginning with systematic desensitization was that it involved first teaching Scott differential relaxation. This was a skill that, even if we did not continue in desensitization, Scott would find very useful in everyday life.

It is interesting to note that the formal assessment of Scott's problem did not extend beyond the first session or two. This was in part due to the pressure of time, but primarily due to my belief that Scott, being a psychologist, would be able to assess his behavior objectively and be able to tell briefly what he was doing in response to what. However, as we found out, this was not entirely the case. While Scott's professional training and experience did help, he was unable, at times, to assess the situation accurately.

The initial therapeutic venture, relaxation training, served several functions. To begin with, it demonstrated Scott's tremendous motivation to be helped and to help himself. Further, it added to Scott's belief that I could help him in ways he could not help himself. Finally, as the initial element in therapy, it made the entire program somewhat successful. I believe that the success of relaxation training in this instance (as well as others) attests to the power of this technique as a therapeutic tool.

At first glance, the work on the development of the hierarchy for desensitization may appear to have been a waste of time. However, I believe it served as a useful if not necessary introduction to what followed. In making up the hierarchy we had to focus on the situations in which Scott became anxious. In particular, Scott had to discriminate between situations and even between elements within a situation. We both became somewhat concerned over our apparent inability to identify crucial elements and differences during this time.

The real problem, however, came when we began systematic desensitization proper. Instead of being able to go through the items in a smooth succession, we kept encountering items that had to be repeated, modified, or added. Further, generalization to the real situation was not going well. It was this frustration with systematic desensitization as well as the discriminations we had begun to make within and between anxiety-provoking situations (along with the early recognition of Scott's perfectionism and self-depreciatory behavior) that brought us as far as the "insight" that came in the seventh session. It is open for question if we could have reached this "insight" more directly or quickly. The conversation and course of the seventh session still cause me to wonder who was the former aphasic. Reading and recalling what transpired, I believe I was exhibiting more problems with my thought processes than Scott. At any rate, aside from getting us on track as to how to proceed, the seventh session proved beyond doubt to me that Scott was just as able as anyone to conceptualize and express his thought.

I make no apologies for what appears to be a degree of confused thinking in that session; the conversation took many directions before it finally got on target. In truth, the elements were all there and it was just a matter of putting them together in the correct arrangement. This arrangement, though, was quite elusive for a while. For example, the possible need for a cathartic experience sounded viable and led us to the notion of trying some kind of modified implosion technique. Although I was getting to the point of being willing to try anything, it just did not fit, either theoretically or empirically.

The key that put the situation back into perspective was Scott's making it clear that the critical element was his fear that perhaps he would *not* recover from his stroke, that he might always be an aphasic. From this it became evident that Scott's anxiety in interpersonal situations was not so much a fear of the situations themselves, but more a fear of them for what they represented; failure in them would reinforce the notion of a permanent loss.

There are implications here that extend beyond this particular situation. We had taken a fairly direct approach to doing systematic desensitization for a fear of interpersonal situations. In developing our hierarchy, we looked for the characteristics of these situations that seemed to cause Scott to become anxious. In doing this, we concerned ourselves with obvious stimuli, such as number of people, degree of acquaintance, etc. in making up the dimensions on which we ordered the items.

With our problems in working through these items in systematic desensitization we realized that these were not the dimensions that were really critical in determining the degree of anxiety experienced by Scott. It was the not-so-obvious dimension of what *failure in these situations* represented to him in terms of reinforcing his belief that he was possibly brain-damaged. It was this "underlying" fear that caused him to be anxious in interpersonal situations. Consequently, the crucial elements in the situation were not concrete stimuli but rather the perceived implications of failure in these situations.

Unlike a "simple" phobia, such as a snake phobia, where there is a single specific phobia object, the kind of "phobia" experienced by Scott appears to be a function of a wide variety of diffuse unconnected stimuli. Apparently, however, there is a common stimulus, given a label by the subject, that unites the situations that give rise to anxiety. Thus, in these cases where one is dealing with this diffuse kind of phobia, it is important to discover not the situational similarities, but the label or stimulus provided by the client. This means looking at the situations from the viewpoint of the client.

By conceptualizing the problem from Scott's perspective, it could not be seen that an *in vivo* approach was needed in which Scott could be given the opportunity to test his label and discover for himself that there was no real basis for his fears. The attack had to be made more directly on his labeling of situations since not only did Scott have to experience success, but he also had to perceive these experiences as successful.

Therapy then took several forms. First, there were the ratings Scott made on his performance. Next were the discussions of what was perception and what was reality. There was the encouragement to give up using props and to become less dependent on them. Scott was advised to read Ellis again. Exposure to more "risky" situations was sought. We discussed the need to focus on the positive aspects of his performance and to pay less attention to the negative. Finally, there was the continued use of differential relaxation to the extent that it could be accomplished by recall.

Happily, all of this seemed to work. For, as Scott notes, he did become more relaxed; he began to perceive his behavior in situations differently; and he began to gain more confidence in his ability to function without props.

Given the change in his behavior over the course of the sessions, I believe we were successful in helping Scott. This is, of course, purely our subjective judgment. However, with the emphasis on perception as opposed to reality, perhaps this is *the* important criteria; at least in this case.

Personally, I appreciate having had the opportunity to work with Scott. It was a positive learning experience for both of us, which is as it should be.

References

Ellis, A., and Harper, R. A. 1963. *A guide to rational living.* Englewood Cliffs, N.J.: Prentice Hall.

Jacobson, E. 1929. *Progressive relaxation.* Chicago: University of Chicago Press.

Moss, C. S. 1969. *Dreams, images, and fantasy: a semantic differential casebook.* Urbana: University of Illinois Press.

Paul, G. L. 1966. *Insight versus desensitization in psychotherapy: an experiment in anxiety reduction.* Stanford: Stanford University Press.

———. 1969. Outcome of systematic desensitization. I-II: Controlled investigations of individual treatment technique variations, and current status. In C. M. Franks (ed.), *Behavior therapy: appraisal and status.* New York: McGraw-Hill.

Reik, T. 1948. *Listening with the third ear.* New York: Farrar, Straus Co.

9

Epilogue

I

While thinking about the stroke sometime after the third anniversary of the incident, I was reminded that it happened on October 30, and that when we moved to Urbana we had thought at long last I would be around to monitor the children on Halloween night, something that because of my heavy travel schedule I had been able to do only once in the previous six years. In light of my accident, it might be construed by some people that there are men who would do almost anything to get out of supervising the kids on trick-or-treat night. In my case they wouldn't be too far wrong.

In January, 1970 I sent a rough copy of part of the manuscript for this book to Joe Wepman to ask his opinions on it and on treatment possibilities. He responded to the latter by stating frankly, "I don't know what else you can do, Scott, beyond what you have already done. Unfortunately, remedial techniques at your level have just never been developed. As you know, most language therapists are equipped to start therapy, but unequipped to follow through at your level. Probably this isn't out of line with my previous comments to you. Your recovery beyond your present state lies almost completely in your hands." I was thankful for his honesty — it confirmed, of course, what my wife and I had already learned.[1]

---

[1] Bette writes: "About a year after the accident Scott got the feeling that

In addition to continuing to teach courses in psychotherapy and community mental health and writing the manuscript of this book (as well as readying two other books for publication), I made two additional formal attempts at therapy, one of which, behavioral therapy, I have already told about in Chapter 8. Simultaneously, I took a course in the psycholinguistics of aphasia. This course was interesting, although the instructor placed a much greater emphasis on the relationship of aphasia to the theory of thought and language and much less on such practical considerations as therapy and re-habilitation, so in this sense it was more of an intellectual endeavor than any emotional confrontation. I had two undergraduate students who signed up to take a course in individual topics with me in the spring semester, and I used them both in reviewing the relevant literature and in my preparation of a term paper on the self-reports of aphasics (Chapter 10).

Even so, despite the joint exercise at further rehabilitation, it seemed clear to us that I could not remain indefinitely in my role as professor. The business of relating to highly intelligent and critical graduate students was just too difficult for me and everyone concerned. By February my correspondence with the mental health coordinator of the federal prison system resulted in the offer of a position to become the chief psychologist at a California prison. This seemed to us to be a viable alternative to remaining at Illinois. It was, for instance, one of the few ways of again becoming a member of the U.S. Public Health Service (which provided the health services to the prison sys-

he wasn't improving. The improvement had slowed because at first it was very rapid; while I still felt there was a lot of improvement every day, he didn't. He asked me to call Dr. Matz, because we were still searching, searching for something else we could do. I think that neither one of us wanted to accept the fact that there wasn't anything else that the medical experts had to offer in terms of therapy, rehabilitation, or medication, anything that would help him to get over the aphasia. Dr. Matz said to me on the phone, 'Do you think there is no more improvement now?' I answered that I didn't feel this way. He responded that if the improvement had absolutely stopped that it might be something to be concerned about, but he couldn't imagine that Scott wasn't still showing some progress. Scott felt better for my having talked with Dr. Matz, but Matz again made it clear that he didn't know anything to recommend for him. I believe we had finally begun to accept that fact, that the experts on aphasia had nothing additional to offer and we were forced back upon our own resources."

tem), without having to travel. While I had never been employed full-time in a correctional institution before, I wasn't completely unfamiliar with correctional programs.

I had once worked part-time for a delinquency program for girls in St. Louis, and when we moved to Fulton, Missouri, the state hospital had contained about 250 "criminally insane" members from the nearby state correctional institution. I had also been an under-utilized consultant to both the men's and women's prisons at Jefferson City. Finally, when I moved to the West Coast as an NIMH consultant, although my main functions were as a mental health generalist and in time as the deputy to the associate director, I also held down the position of regional representative of the crime and delinquency branch of the Institute. In this job I had extended contacts with the leading correctional authorities in each of the western states. Specifically, my work related to research projects, both adult and juvenile, with a heavy emphasis placed on prevention or re-habilitation through community programs.

I had a number of other reasons for accepting the appointment in a federal correctional institution, ranging all the way from social and humanitarian reasons down to the most private, some of which I have already mentioned. In this particular era there was a tremendous emphasis on "law and order" which had come to prevail in the criminal justice system and in society as a whole, and in which I was naturally concerned as a socially oriented psychologist. I was struck with the fact that the structure of the prison system was roughly like that of state hospitals twenty-five to thirty years ago, and I felt that perhaps I could make contributions based on some of the things that we profited from and some of the mistakes we had made in the mental health system.

Most important, there were a whole host of private reasons, such as the fact that I would become eligible automatically for federal group life insurance, from which I had been cut off by my oversight in not taking out life insurance as a professor, before my accident. Last and most important, the prison represented an escape for me, a getting out of the competitive professional life, a chance to hide behind the tall gray walls and join the inmates in their forced retirement, but with a compensation. As an allied staff member of the Department of Justice,

I would collect retirement at a third faster rate than ordinary, i.e., receiving three years' retirement for each two worked. These latter reasons were naturally calculated to place my family in its most secure financial position.

In early April, I met with Don Peterson and informed him of our pending decision to return to federal service. I think we were both relieved at the decision; however, as would be expected, he spoke mostly of his hope that the new position would be beneficial to me. I mentioned that I would be most anxious in the first six months, since this was my probationary period in federal service, at which juncture he volunteered that I should not think of resigning from the university, but instead ask for a six months' leave of absence. I had never considered this and hadn't known that it was a possibility; however, I responded to the suggestion with warm thanks, and indicated that I would talk with the chairman about it. As it turned out, Mort Weir, like Don, was most accepting of the arrangement, and said he would carry my letter of request to the higher administrative officials. In very short order the leave of absence was arranged. The university was exceedingly kind and understanding under very unfortunate circumstances for everyone concerned.

Before the decision was finally made, I went to Decatur to see a young neurosurgeon who had been highly recommended by our nurse friend, Mary Nolte. I liked him at once. He was extremely knowledgeable and very honest in discussing the problem with me. I had several questions to ask him, including whether he would give me an independent assessment of my condition; whether I should be taking any medication; and what he thought medically of my taking another position. We talked for about forty minutes and he ended by giving me yet another thorough physical examination.

Throughout the conversation the surgeon kept referring to my condition as stemming from a "disease," which was contrary to the way that I had always thought about my accident. I felt called upon to inquire into his use of the term. There was no mistake about his regarding my type of stroke as attributable to a disease brought about by several decades of luxurious eating habits. He cited the fact that Americans are succumbing to circulatory disorders at an increasingly early age and that cross-culturally many other recently developing countries were now attempting to emulate the lamentable record of the United States. He also indicated that the youngest patient whom he had seen was thirty-seven, so my having a stroke at age forty-three was not a record.

Another thing that I learned from our conversation was that my left internal carotid artery was totally clogged. As it turned out, the neurosurgeons at Presbyterian–St. Luke's had discovered this by the use of the angiogram, but had failed to communicate it in such a way that it was understandable to Bette and hence to me. Because of my relatively excellent recovery, I had fantasied that possibly only one division of the internal carotid artery was blocked (perhaps only the central division similar to Rose's affliction, p. 188). Instead, this physician attributed my recovery to the supporting circulation system stemming from the right carotid. He stated that he was frankly surprised at my almost complete recovery in that there is an inverse relationship between age and recovery when the entire carotid artery is blocked, that is, when one of the arteries in older people slowly clogs over time, it gives the other-sided artery time to maximize the increased circulation; this seldom happens in people as young as myself, and ends most frequently with disastrous results.[2]

These were his seven concrete recommendations:

(1) There would be no role for a neurosurgeon such as himself unless I began developing additional symptoms which indicated that the right carotid artery or the supporting network that emanated from

---

[2] When the internal carotid artery became permanently clogged, it hypothetically could have cut off most of the circulation to my dominant cerebral hemisphere, thus subjecting me to partial paralysis, bilateral hemianesthesia, blindness, and aphasia. However, as it became gradually apparent to me from studying books on neurophysiology, blood flows from the external carotid into the ophthalamic artery, which may become a source of circulation when the internal carotid is occluded. Another source of auxillary circulation is the Circle of Willis, which is a polygonal arrangement of blood vessels at the base of the brain. The Circle of Willis is frequently the site of developmental defects, but in my case one would assume that these two sources of collateral circulation have held up fairly well thus far. It is important that the flow of blood be kept constant, which may account in part for the fact that even today I seem to have fluctuations in performance. I think of myself as essentially similar to people who function with one lung or one kidney, except my capacity for speech and/or memory is more-or-less permanently impaired.

it was beginning to fail, e.g., such signs as partial blindness or numbness of either side since the side affected is unpredictable.

(2) I should get a qualified neurosurgeon who could check me periodically. It might have been taken for granted, but believe it or not, this was the first time any physician had given me such counsel.

(3) He strongly urged that I should go on a near-starvation diet, since he was worried about not only further cerebral complications but possible cardiac involvement.

(4) He would not recommend any medication, and he spoke disparagingly of oral anticoagulants, including, incidentally, the medication that I had taken for eight months (among the side effects of that particular drug he listed possible depressive reactions).

(5) He had nothing but praise for my keeping as physically active as possible, including the fact that I was then engaged in lugging very heavy stones into my back yard from surrounding building sites for aesthetic reasons.

(6) I should drink very heavily of fluids (as a blood thinner), and I should learn to drink liquor in moderation (as a vasodilator) — advice for which I thanked him, since it was contrary to my expectations.

(7) On the basis of my physical exam, which again yielded nothing negative, he counseled no objection to taking another position that might be somewhat easier for me, and in fact volunteered that there was no need even to mention that I had had a stroke unless I felt called upon to be strictly honest, since it was undetectable without elaborate tests.

At this juncture I should add one other point:

(8) My faith in physicians in general and neurosurgeons in particular was restored by this contact. A long time before, through my contact with colleagues, either psychiatrists or psychologists, I had learned one must carefully scrutinize the clinician before making a commitment to him. My anxiety had dissipated to the point where I could begin to differentiate and to recognize again that obviously doctors, like members of any other profession, are only human beings, too.

One other thing that bears note: during the meeting the surgeon said that he was afraid of making me into a neurotic by reciting the symptoms of which I should be aware. I laughingly assured him that I couldn't become more neurotic than I already was; however, the meeting did serve to alarm my wife. In playing the tape which I had dutifully made on my hidden recorder, she became very concerned about my welfare, and became even more highly solicitous than usual in the next few days. Within a week her concern became further evidenced, in that she became suddenly aware that her heart was skipping beats. When I inquired into her obvious dismay, she described herself as fearful of some impending catastrophe, but she could not (or would not) identify the object.

Ten days later Bette became so highly anxious that we made a hurried visit to an internist, who took an EKG. Afterwards he spoke to her candidly, saying that there was no reason to be alarmed about her condition, since many people suffer from asymptomatic heartbeats, and it was not indicative of any developing heart disorder. This seemed to partly mollify her, but for the next couple of weeks, on going to bed she would go through a ritual, inquiring about the "gushiness' of the blood in my right artery, and I would, in turn, ask whether her heart was still pumping regularly.

Bette wrote then about my rehabilitation and our decision to move back into federal service:

"The stroke has happened and as much as I try to repress it, every once in a while when we'd talk in the last year, Scott would say such things as 'I can't lecture any more, it's too difficult,' and 'I can't do this and I can't do that.' I'd try to minimize them, but perhaps this wasn't good, because he would end up getting angry with me. I wanted to convince him that other people didn't look at him the same way he looked at himself. He finally did convince me, in part. When he had to prepare his lectures word by word, and I would see the strain on him when he came home from lecturing, nobody would have agreed that this is what he should have been doing. And yet I think that neither of us wanted to give up just yet. We saw him get better in so many other respects, but I felt that anything we could do that would be easier on him would be what we should do. So this is what prompted us to look around. Moving is really incidental. The point that I tried to make is that Scott's work should be satisfying to him, and we could adjust to almost anything. Good Lord, if we could adjust to Illinois we could adjust to any place (except maybe Alaska, which for some reason always struck Scott's fancy). So this prompted our inquiries again.

"There are many factors for not liking it here — just the fact that the accident happened so soon after coming here may be the largest single factor. We want to get out of this place, we want to forget about it. It's been hard on all of us. Maybe it has given us a better understanding of each other, maybe it has brought our family closer together, but this is one heck of a way to do it. . . .

"I am very relieved to be leaving the members of the medical profession here, and I hope to live some place where we can be in touch with competent neurologists. I think that we both agree that we are no longer attracted to university life, and we don't like the setup here — behavioral mod is a drag as far as I'm concerned. It's hard for Scott and would have been difficult even if he hadn't had the accident. So I think our decision to move and get out of here and to make a new life again in California is the best thing that we could do.

"I think if this is as far as the improvement goes, if what we have left now is still some aphasia so that it causes him to block now and then, this we can live with and he can still maintain a professional practice. Everything else, though, to me, is quite normal about Scott. The one thing that I have noticed recently is the return of his sense of humor. This was the slowest thing to come back. Perhaps he thought these things but he didn't say them, especially where two or three people were present. He picked up on what someone else said that was humorous, but he didn't make these comments that he was so adept at making before. But now he has begun to do this again. . . . I don't think improvement is at a standstill even yet. . . ."

In former moments of despair, I used to say to Bette, "If only I could function as a psychologist and not be called upon to relate to people," which is an ironic comment for a clinician. For the first time in my adult life, I fit the old saying, "A man not interested in his work is like a frog under a drag." But as time went on the obstacles and the resulting despondency gave way to a fairly reasoned and more articulate perception of the situation.

In a very real sense every one of my professional activities is a form of therapy for me. My primary observable deficit is the inability to communicate with myself and others, and therefore a large part of all of my professional activities is self-directed rehabilitation. Whether I am teaching a formal class, directing students in the conduct of psychotherapy, sitting down to discuss individual topics, directing dissertations, arguing on a subject with my colleagues, dictating correspondence to Bette, trying to train Julie or Kevin in some phase of school work, simply in pounding the keys of the typewriter, or attempting to get across what it is like to be an aphasic — each of my interpersonal responsibilities calls upon intricate forms of com-munication and is therefore a form of self-therapy — though I really didn't recognize it at the beginning.

II

The move back to California went smoothly enough at the end of the 1970 summer semester. We lived for seven weeks in a motel awaiting the construction of a large Spanish-style home on an acre of ground in a rural setting. I went into debt even further to purchase the house. Other than the change in jobs, we very deliberately made no other concession to my malady — the financial pressures almost made it mandatory that I succeed.

One may wonder at this strategy, but the whole tactic was *not* to give in to the concept that I was an "ill" or "sick" or a "handicapped" person who would trade upon his disease for solace or sympathy. After several earlier transitory attempts at "normal" role-playing in the old setting, in this new situation it became a deadly serious act. This is the reason why I did not tell anyone in the new setting about my stroke, except for the coordinator of mental health in Washington. Incidentally, I recognize this as a direct expression of the behavior theory that I had been partially impressed with. A society's tendency to label people who it supposedly wants to help can produce more of the very deviant behavior which it hopes to extinguish. Take for example the individual who because of some test results is labeled mentally retarded. Other people begin acting toward him as if he were a very slow learner and it takes but a short time before he begins to validate their hypothesis. The patient perceives himself to be mentally retarded and acts, and is reinforced for acting, accordingly.

I was impressed with the level of staff competence that I met at the Federal Correctional Institution (especially the warden); however, the job of rehabilitating the 1,200 inmates left me highly ambivalent, as I recognized the fact that the FCI is not in any sense a mirror image of the community. It is a prison first and foremost, devoted to the protection of society. It represented a wide, almost insurmountable, schism between the closed community of the correctional system and the open society. In the final analysis, of course, it is the fault of the communities themselves for disavowing the responsibility for the care and rehabilitation of the inmates (much as it was for more than a hundred years in this country with the mental patient and the state hospitals). However, my dream about escaping into the prison turned out to be totally unreal. The warden had plans for the activation of a new, progressive "human relations center" which embodied many community mental health principles. I was to be the head of it as the director of mental health. Over a period of several months the mental health staff was increased from two psychologists to seven professional people, three consultants, and a half-dozen graduate students in training.

My interest in research was not neglected either. Shortly after we returned I was contacted by the regional office of NIMH and asked if I would occasionally act as a consultant for it; then the California Department of Mental Hygiene in Sacramento sent a letter requesting that I be a member of their state research advisory committee, and finally, my old friend Ed Glaser asked me to be a consultant for the Human Interaction Research Institute, an organization that specializes in research utilization. In addition, one of the new Ph.D. psychologists who was hired by FCI was research-oriented, as was one of the three consultants, and both were behaviorists. I became involved with one of the consultants in writing a book on training psychological counselors in the correctional setting (Hosford and Moss, forthcoming).

A month or so after our arrival here I came down with a cold, which was unusual for me, particularly since the accident. In preceding years the children had invariably contracted the colds first and then had incubated them like the little test tubes that they were, before passing them onto their parents, but I have been unusually resistant to respiratory infections in the past three years. Anyway, it was no better or worse than any other cold except that it left me with a nagging cough. The pressure of the new position had already got to me and each evening I fell into an exhausted sleep and each morning awoke at 4 or 4:30 and lay in bed mentally preparing for the coming day's events.

The cough and the insomnia were reminiscent of the days immediately preceding my stroke, so this time I wasn't at all reluctant, as I had been previously, to see an internist in Santa Barbara. He diagnosed the cough as due to a postnasal drip and gave me medication to arrest it. He also speculated that there was indeed a relationship between my coughing and the occurrence of the cerebrovascular accident. To wit, the coughing interrupts the flow of blood from the heart and repeated seizures of violent and prolonged choking could cause a clot to form which might be caught in an already narrowed artery. Rightly or not my wife and I felt a momentary vindication in our assumption that my cold had some instigating effect with the resulting accident.

When I made the transition from Illinois to California I of course brought with me the strong recommendation that I place myself in the hands of a competent neurologist who would be in a position to assist me if and when any emergency situation arose. After some inquiry I settled upon a neuropsychiatrist also in Santa Barbara. As it turned out he was an exceedingly competent professional person who took the tack that while his services would be available if I felt the need to call upon him, he would feel much better prepared if I would commit myself to a thorough examination in a local hospital and have a "base rate" established which could provide a benchmark that we could check on annually. This I did, undergoing a complete inspection, including skull films, X-rays of the skull and chest, a blood work-up, a complete neurophysiological and psychological examination, and a painstaking investigation by the internist.

The results were as follows: (1) the examination revealed me to be in generally excellent physical shape; (2) as far as could be determined without subjecting me to the danger of a repeat angiogram, the circulation was completely restored in the left hemisphere, which, in turn, led to the speculation that perhaps the internal carotid artery had reopened (this apparently does happen in about 20 percent of the cases); and (3) they found that I had diabetes. The neuropsychiatrist was quite excited over the last discovery and felt that this could have been the causative factor in my stroke. Like more than a million other Americans, I had developed a mild, adult-onset diabetes, and diabetics are prone to develop vascular complications. Specifically, he spoke of a fat platelet that could have broken free and been caught by a congenitally injured artery — although it was all hypothetical, of course. My condition was assessed as only a moderate case of diabetes which could be controlled by diet and oral antidiabetic drugs, thus for the moment allowing me to escape from having to take insulin injections.

Actually, I wasn't too surprised at the diagnosis. I had suspected for some years that my habit of substituting sweets for regular meals might at some point get me into serious difficulties, although once again the doctors maintain that this has nothing to do with the formation of diabetes. As I have already related, in 1966, when I had difficulties with my eyesight, "George," the prior internist, had run some blood tests which indicated that I had some difficulty assimilating sugar. He had laid down a diet for me which I promptly forgot when the symptom cleared up. Recently, I had become aware of the increasing frequency of urination, especially when I made the move to the prison where toilets for staff members were at a premium. Admittedly there is no direct cause-and-effect evidence linking vascular difficulty with derangement of carbohydrate metabolism, i.e., vascular lesions continue to develop even in the best controlled diabetes. The possibility exists that both may be only a reflection of over-rapid aging.

Those findings of the psychological examination which focused on intellectual functioning were of special interest to me since the tests were objective evidence of my performance. The following examiner's report describes the results:

[The] request for an evaluation of the intellectual functioning of Dr. Moss was an interesting challenge. He holds an American Board Diploma in clinical psychology so might be expected to be thoroughly conversant with the most popular tests for evaluating mental efficiency and organicity. I employed the Bender Gestalt and Memory for Designs tests because familiarity with them would not help a person whose perceptual-motor skills were severely damaged. He did very well on both of these tests. His perceptual ability is not impaired and his coordination is normal.

The Air Force Perception Test demonstrated superior perceptual integration ability.

The Babcock Test fell into disuse when it was replaced with the Wechsler Test so Dr. Moss was not familiar with it. The Babcock Test showed that Dr. Moss had about 75% of his original efficiency in learning new material and motor skills. Part of this loss of efficiency can be attributed to normal, expected age changes. His efficiency was 40%, which is pathologically poor, in repeating digits forward and in reverse order. He had 70% efficiency in recalling sentences from memory. He remembers well facts he has learned and anything to which he can apply his superior reasoning ability. Repeating numbers, where there is no logical sequence, is difficult for him. He is better in recalling sentences because they have meaning.

The Slosson Intelligence Test was unfamiliar to Dr. Moss so it was employed to evaluate his overall intellectual functioning. On this test, he earned IQ 140. He had failures at age 10, 11 and 12 on Memory for Digits. His four highest successes were tests of vocabulary, information and arithmetic problem-solving. In arithmetic problem-solving, his mathematical logic is unimpaired but his speed of manipulation of numbers is extremely slow. Computations which require 15 seconds normally kept Dr. Moss busy for 1½ to 2 minutes.

Dr. Moss said that word-finding, memory and arithmetic are current problems for him. He finds it difficult to talk before a group without copious notes because he may block and be unable to proceed.[3]

The report of the psychologist indicated, as I had expected, that I suffered no perceptual motor loss, and my coordination and perceptual ability were unimpaired. Vocabulary, information, mathematical problem-solving, and conceptualizing verbal relationships (unintentionally omitted from the report) were scored as the highest successes. It was in gross learning of new information that I suffered the greatest loss, particularly the rote memorization of new, logically unrelated facts, e.g., memory for digits forwards and backwards. My arithmetical ability remained intact although I found it exceedingly difficult to keep the numbers in mind to compute with; thus on an untimed test I could reason my way through to a correct answer, but for all intents I could no longer compute effectively.

On the other side of the ledger, I was elated to learn, about this

[3]Robert L. Brigden, Ph.D., letter to Hal C. Gregg, M.D., January 23, 1971.

time, that my recent book, *Dreams, Images, and Fantasy,* had been selected for distribution by a professional book club. Using this one standard criterion of acceptance, I scored satisfactorily for someone who has had to combat a stroke and the residuals of aphasia.

Bette has been naturally very happy being back in sunny California and our three children seem to have made friends quickly and become established in their new schools. It is difficult to be objective about what effect my accident has had on the children. I am comparatively quiet relative to what I used to be and I continue to make word errors, especially when I am tired or upset, but I think that they have adjusted all-in-all to my speaking idiosyncrasies.

III

In summary, it really was a potentially tragic experience that befell us almost four years ago. It seems to us that everything went against us, in that we had just moved to a new community, we had few friends there, we had to make decisions with a basic lack of information, we were in a city that apparently didn't have a good specialist, or perhaps in our extreme anxiety no one would have sufficed, but the result was that nowhere along the line did we feel that we received any really adequate advice.

What was needed at the beginning were a couple of extended conversations with a neurologist in whom we had confidence, who would tell us what was wrong with me, what had happened along the way, and what was likely to happen in the future. If a physician had seen me early in the illness, he would doubtlessly have been quite pessimistic at my serious initial handicap (most likely predicting that I would never recover anywhere near full functioning of my language), but if he continued with me after the first couple of months then he would have been afraid to predict, probably leaving the prognosis up in the air (which is the way we would have wanted it, since each recovered function came as a pleasant surprise).

It wasn't too surprising that the neurosurgeons at Chicago didn't do more in the way of rehabilitation. As I have come to recognize, neurosurgeons are a specialized breed, whose main interest is in neurology quite removed from the behavioral issues. They are interested in the "dynamics" of the circulatory system (why it was that my collateral circulation was so great), quite removed from my psychological dynamics. I have come to accept that their interest was restricted to my nervous system and was not in me as a human being.

When I returned from Chicago with not a single professional person in the community to help out, it is impressive that my wife survived the experience. It was all so terribly frightening to have this happen to any family. We were simply thrown back into the home, almost totally on our own resources. Thank goodness that we latched onto the university speech clinic for the counseling and supportive therapy that they gave us. Yet I don't look on my experience as being too atypical of the way most aphasics are treated. Obviously we needed some professional help, but given the circumstances it is not clear to me what move my wife or I could have made that would have improved the situation.

We never did receive even the booklets dealing with aphasia prepared by the heart/stroke/speech/ or rehabilitation people, which I subsequently found out about. These give all sorts of minor, practical advice, such as, to the wife, "You mustn't treat him as a child because that will make him mad," or "Just because your husband doesn't talk well, don't think that he is stupid." They go on to state that intelligence is not affected, which of course is not true, but it doubt-lessly makes for better motivation all the way around. They also give advice about trying to perform therapy for the patient. The point is that physicians should have some awareness that these pamphlets do exist and make them available to their patients. It is really such a minor thing to ask; it does appear that so little effort could have helped a lot.

Of course, my wife and I began to take steps, faltering as they may have been, to regain as much of my verbal and intellectual competence as soon as we could. I have no doubt that if my wife had not been able to give so completely of herself in my early recovery, I would not have regained my abilities nearly to this extent — it would have been easier to have settled for much less. And the fact that I have always been such a perfectionist certainly relates to my unceasing drive to get well. It is true, my self-imposed high standards made me hyper-sensitive about my disabilities, real or imagined; on the other hand, they made me strive mightily to get over them. In the period of three years plus, I have overcome some of my early deficiencies and compensated for others, although I have to admit that a few handicaps defeated our best efforts.

Looked at in retrospect, I have a strong hunch that the artery began to close some time ago, six months, a year, twenty years before the stroke, or maybe the walls of the artery have always had a congenital defect — what else could have prepared the left hemisphere to make the transition to the blood supply emanating from the right artery? For what other reason would I have suffered such a relatively mild aphasia and thought disorganization with relatively rapid recovery from a really major stroke?

Looking back over the first forty-five months after the accident, I must admit that the most dramatic recovery took place within the first six months, but with the qualification that I continued to reacquire more subtle capacities all the time. By 1971 I still suffered from a very spotty memory and a resultant loss of word-finding. Contrary to the prediction advanced much earlier that given time my speaking difficulty would disappear, it remains at this writing uppermost in every interaction that I have. As long as I relate to a single individual, the interaction goes fairly smoothly; as the size of the group increases and/or my role becomes more prominent and/or the discussion turns to the abstract, then my ability (and confidence) decreases.

On the other hand, I can still get up and give a formal presentation if I can plan ahead and can actually have the lecture in front of me. In a very real sense, I suppose this was predictable even before the stroke. Most people have difficulty under these circumstances and I was no exception, except that now the problem of communicating is grossly magnified. I used to feel anxious when I was slated to play a prominent role in a large meeting where I was expected to interact spontaneously; now I am subtly concerned in any relationship whatsoever, fearful I may give expression to my deficiencies. This still includes almost any situation outside of my immediate family. But I am also convinced now that most of the remaining problems are inside, concerned with the recapturing of memories or thought difficulties; nevertheless, I have learned largely to disguise the outward manifestation.

Sometimes I have found myself thinking that this may be my last book, since I am told that this type of health problem is apparently very unpredictable — that in the next moment I may have another such accident. I do feel fortunate in completing this manuscript, which makes three books that I theoretically should not have written. But I also remember Lordet (Riese, p. 240) and the fact that he lived forty-five years after his stroke (dying at the age of ninety-eight), and that he was professionally productive much of that time — so it does happen. Even more than that, it has been extremely providential to be able to achieve a postponement to settle my affairs, an accomplishment that is denied to many people.

As I struggled to recover, I remember thinking that if aphasia happens to the average working man, in a sense it isn't as bad, at least the poor fellow isn't attempting to make a living with words. In time I came to realize that this was one more exercise in self-pity; obviously the typical stroke victim does suffer some degree of permanent paralysis so his manner of making a living is similarly affected. After the stroke I attempted to hide from other people the fact that I had ever suffered such an accident, but finally I have come to realize that I must accept myself as I am. I cannot be deceitful and maintain that it has not been a constant, daily struggle, and in the process I have learned the meaning of human frailty. Yet my family has survived and prospered, I am alive, and for the most part, all things considered, I do very well.

References

Hosford, R., and Moss, C. S. *The crumbling walls: treatment and counseling of the youthful offender* (in preparation).

Riese, W. 1954. Auto-observation reported by eminent nineteenth century medical scientist. *Bulletin of Historical Medicine,* 28, 237-242.

10

A Review of the
Self-Reports of Aphasics

About the turn of the new year in 1970, I called Professor William Brewer to inquire whether he would allow me to audit his course in psycholinguistics and aphasia, since it would provide me with an opportunity to acquire more information about aphasia and learn what, if anything, I could do about additional treatment. He knew vaguely of my recent history and welcomed me to the class, which consisted of a small group of students who were expected to participate fully in the proceedings. The content was almost exclusively theoretical, however, and was hardly at all about what could be done about the condition. (Bill was skeptical about there being any formal, effective therapy for the aphasic on the limited information available.) Intellectually the course was pitched at an advanced level that exceeded my very limited professional background, but Bill was understanding and placed no demands upon me. I was further disadvantaged because while I had been a practicing clinician for two decades, I hadn't until very recently ever seen anyone except myself that I would classify as an aphasic. Almost all such cases are routinely sent to speech therapists rather than to psychologists.

I chose as my topic a review of journal articles and books that dealt with the self-reports of aphasics. I eventually gave my review before the class.[1] I took on my assignment enthusiastically since, as far as I

---

[1] I have kept this chapter basically in the form it was when I wrote it in

know, such a survey hadn't been given before, at least it hadn't appeared in print. More important, my idea that self-treatment was the only way to combate the residuals seemed to be confirmed. Bill and I kept secret the fact that I had had a stroke and that I was an aphasic in good remission. I took delight in attempting to keep to the role of a normal person over time, although there were many times in the class when I might have confessed. Insofar as I am aware, the other students will first learn that I had inside information on aphasia when they perchance read this book.

A recent Illinois Ed.D., Irene Ostoff, wrote her thesis on a particular aspect of how to train counselors (1970). I was a member of her committee. She selected schizophrenia as a topic that most educational counselors knew little about, and introduced it to beginning graduate students by having them read the regular college texts written by professional workers along with literary accounts, many of them self-reports written by former schizophrenics. She found that either way served as an introduction to the subject, that is, both groups of students profited from the experience through an increased understanding of how to interact with such patients. So, too, did I profit from the exposure to articles by aphasics. Certainly I was able to identify and empathize to a greater extent with persons who had suffered cortical injury, and I learned that my personal experience was not too different from the majority of those expressed by other stroke victims.

There are nine articles and five books in the English language that I managed to identify. I will approach the literature more or less chronologically, dealing first with the journal articles. The main focus wherever possible will be the degree of recovery that was evidenced and to what the individuals attributed their rehabilitation.

I. Reports of Journal Articles

Let us begin with the illustrious Samuel Johnson. Johnson was seventy-three and in poor health when he suffered a stroke in the

---

May of 1970 as a report to Brewer's class; as such it is representative of my progress at that time. Appreciation is extended to two of my students, J. Isaac Levy and Richard L. Block, for their assistance in reviewing and discussing this literature with me.

middle of the night in 1783 (Critchley, 1962). He awoke and immediately realized what had happened. There was no paralysis aside from a temporary facial asymmetry, but fearing for his sanity, he executed a prayer in Latin, and being satisfied that his intellect was intact, he fell back asleep again. The next morning he discovered that he could not talk but could write letters with some difficulty. His disability continued throughout the ensuing days but in diminishing severity, so that by the end of the week there remained little loss of facility in language.

Critchley presents photographs of a series of letters written by Johnson, beginning with the first day and continuing until the fifty-seventh day of his illness. Perusal of them reveals a general untidines᷉ of penmanship, numerous instances of verbal corrections, even a possible neologism or two, but no real loss in vocabulary. A gross statistical analysis of his phraseology revealed no striking difference in those written before and those after the stroke. His physician treated him with blisters of the head and throat.

Johnson died eighteen months later. His right kidney was removed and preserved by the postmortem attendant, but no one thought to preserve his remarkable brain. Critchley states three reasons why the aphasia was not severe and comparatively short in duration: (1) the pathological lesion might have been small in size; (2) the very magnitude of Johnson's literary capacity might have exercised a beneficial effect in restoring his linguistic function, and (3) he might have been left-handed and therefore no frank unilateral cerebral dominance existed.

The second report was by Jean de Fouchy, seventy-seven, formerly the permanent secretary of the French Academy of Science (Hoff et al., 1958). He was walking home alone one night in 1824 when he tripped, hitting his head on a stone. The next day, during dinner, he became unable to pronounce the words that he wanted to speak. He heard what was said, he was not paralyzed, but he was simply unable to use the words that would express his thoughts. The episode lasted about one minute.

The next year, 1825, Jacques Lordat, a prominent member of the medical school of Montpellier, suffered a stroke (Riese, 1954). He was fifty-three at the time. His impairment came on gradually over twenty-four hours, he suffered no coma nor any paralysis, but he suffered both an expressive and a receptive impediment. That is, all but a few words eluded his grasp, and he could not fit those that remained into a sentence; he also was aware that he could no longer grasp what other people were saying — they spoke too rapidly for him to grasp their meaning. That was true for reading as well as speaking.

He felt that his "inner speech" was unimpaired because he made up lectures in his head and therefore couldn't believe that he was ill, but as soon as anyone came to see him, he again became aware of his complete inability to say anything. This led Lordat to recognize the importance of language in conserving, preserving, and transmitting ideas, but it also led him to the observation that verbal signs were not indispensable or even necessary for thought. "I was in full possession of the inner aspect [of thought], having lost [only] its external manifestations." So his outstanding contribution was that thought and language are neither identical nor parallel.

After some weeks of deep melancholy, it dawned on him that he could suddenly read the title of a book. Though the process was slow, "I made use of this faculty to re-educate myself in speaking and writing." Unfortunately, he did not describe the specific measures used. Lordat termed the episode "verbal amnesia" and coined the term of "paramesia" for the faulty use of words (i.e., substituting "handkerchief" for "book," etc.). Lordat resumed being a teacher, and lived until ninety-eight. Riese lists nineteen major papers, including fourteen written after Lordat's recovery from aphasia.

In 1948 a physician named Rose published his account of a thrombosis of the left middle cerebral artery which he sustained in 1943 at the age of sixty-eight. He, too, did not suffer any paralysis and reported that while he understood every sentence spoken to him, he could not say a single word. Rose was hospitalized for five months. He tried to keep his mind occupied ("otherwise I couldn't stand it") and for the first two years he played the radio constantly. Within four months he began to say a few words and during the year his speech gradually improved. He reported, "I get practice from reading, from the radio and from the movies." He could write with difficulty and do simple arithmetic, but had lost the ability to read.

At a YMCA he joined a group who enjoyed song fests, and this brought the discovery that he could sing all of the old songs perfectly.

This led, in turn, to his perception of what seemed to be a relationship between memorization and the secret of learning to talk again. Rose reasoned that the brain pathway for singing is parallel with that for memorization. He then proceeded, in an immense amount of time, to learn the Lord's Prayer, the 23rd Psalm, "Crossing the Bar," and finally "Thanatopsis." "My speech took a great forward spurt, I seemed to gain as much in one week as I had previously in three months. . . . The speechless one was talking freely." He then wrote a treatise on *Memorization as an Aid in the Treatment of Aphasia* three years after the stroke. Rose postulated that "in this way you can enlarge your vocabulary to any extent that you may wish."

Wendell Johnson, then editor of the *Journal of Speech and Hearing Disorders,* heard about Rose's paper and eventually had it published. In an unintentional humorous footnote Johnson sent Dr. Rose a copy of his newly published book, *People in Quandries.* Rose responded that he tried to read it, but it was "almost my Nemesis . . . I bit off more than I could chew. I certainly would have risked another stroke or some vascular accident if I had followed through. I did not realize that my trouble was confined so definitely in the reading and writing areas."

Next came two reports by former enlisted servicemen, one in the Army and the other in the Navy. They were the first recipients of modern treatment techniques. Alonzo Hall was involved in an automobile accident during the last days of the war with Japan. His condition was diagnosed as "Concussion, cerebral, and contusion, left temporoparietal area, manifested by paresis. Secondary diagnosis: Aphasia, reflex changes, and deformity of skull, bilateral." He was "unconscious" for three weeks and eight months later was released from service and given 100 percent disability benefits.

Hall (1961) began his speech therapy while still in an Army hospital and was taught sound movements and techniques designed to help a stutterer deal with feelings induced by social penalties. Feelings of anxiety developed and within six months he was excused from speech clinic activities and subsequently discharged from the Army. On the outside, he entered a university speech clinic, which did nothing for his halting speech but after eight months did bring him to his first dawning acceptance of his limitations and strengths. He then returned home, but his disabilities, while seemingly accepted by his friends and family, served only to reinforce his own self-rejection.

Hall next enrolled in a business college and took courses in penmanship, typing, spelling, and arithmetic. The silences persisted in his speech and the distortions in his gait were still evident. He then enrolled in the university, and upon completion of his degree he noted that his rate of speech was increased, his writing was more legible, and his gait approached normality. Unfortunately, his speech was still inadequate for successful competition on the job market. He was finally guided into psychotherapy. As a result of therapy, socially acceptable skills replaced his withdrawal from society and his perceptions of self were made more objective. Hall concluded that psychotherapy helps perceptual distortions and that then the patient can make greater strides toward recovery in conventional speech therapy.

The second report is somewhat parallel with the first. In 1955 Dick Butler was in a motorcycle accident and suffered a head injury. He was twenty years old at the time, was hospitalized for eight months, and was discharged from the Navy with a 100 percent disability rating. His article (Sies and Butler, 1963) is an account of what ensued for the next six years.

Upon discharge, Butler returned home. He found the world unmanageable, was painfully aware of his many deficiencies, and withdrew into himself. Two years after the accident, he enrolled at a university, but found mathematics too abstract, physics and zoology too tedious, and even the social sciences not really satisfying. He then dropped from school for one semester, only to find that the school would not accept him back. Nevertheless, he established contact with a speech therapist at the university, and began a series of interviews in which he drew upon his thoughts and feelings as an aphasic.

Let me paraphrase some of the insights into how an aphasic such as Butler interprets his world: My greatest difficulty in speaking resides in my subvocal grouping and repeated self-corrections. My memory is a revolving card file of experience and in order to recall something, this card file must revolve until a pattern or image begins to take form and is represented by words in my vocabulary. Too often my tabula rosa remains blank. That is, I must first get a clear signal; then as I conceptualize the referent, I choose the words for what I hope will be effective communication. But the process is short-circuited — the circuits of thought remain incomplete (difficulty in conceptualization), or a blockage may occur in word-choosing interfering with clear and appropriate verbal language for effectual expression (difficulties in language). Then if I have still not made myself understood, I begin frantically "reaching for" and putting together more words in which to make my meaning clearer, that is, if the meaning is still clear to me. But often I can't recall an appropriate word or phrase and I respond to any misinterpretation by frowning, grimacing, or banging the table. I suffer ungracefully when I find a hole in my map.

Finally, we came to two other papers, the first entitled "Aphasia as seen by the aphasic." Rolnick and Hoops (1970) interviewed six mild aphasics and systematically reported on their reactions to problems on comprehension, expression, reading, writing, and family reaction. They came up with such points as the following: in comprehension of speech, the speaker should slow down the rate of speech and not make his sentences too involved, and similarly, the process of expression seems to be slowed down in the aphasic. The second paper is "A glimpse into an aphasic's world," written by a neophyte occupational therapy worker, Albertson (1947). It is a somewhat charming account of one student's brush with aphasia and makes optimistic suggestions to what occupational therapy may accomplish.

II. Books Written by or about Aphasics

Now we come to a spate of five books, all written in the past decade. I will give just a word or two by way of introduction. All of the books detail the frankly alarming experience of what it is like to go through the stroke and the long, frustrating efforts at some semblance of rehabilitation. The stroke itself isn't that bad, at least for the patient. The temporal sequence is characterized by the abrupt onset and rapid evolution, and the symptoms usually reach a peak of severity in seconds or minutes. It is largely painless (brains are numb — they know only what the body experiences). The patient may react with momentary anxiety but the initial phase almost always is characterized by varying degrees of clouding of consciousness with confusion, disorientation, and the occurrence of altered forms of symbolic expression. A severe stroke may result in loss of consciousness, complete paralysis, global aphasia, and in one out of ten cases, death. It really is not a bad way to die, if one has any choice in the matter. But what follows if the patient lives (and the great majority of them do) is not at all a pleasant story.

Doug Ritchie (1966) was fifty years old when he suffered a stroke. He worked for the British Information Services of BBC. He characterized his premorbid personality as being moody, ambitious, worrisome, not too verbose, and definitely influenced by the opinions of others. He classified himself as an introvert. He had also suffered from high blood pressure for five to six years before the stroke. When the stroke occurred he ended up in a comatose state in a nursing home for four days, and remained there for almost eight weeks before he went home in the care of his wife.

When Ritchie awoke from the coma he found that he could neither speak nor write and that the right side of his body was paralyzed, but he thought his mind was not affected. It is noteworthy that his paralysis and inability to speak did not concern him — he was convinced that he would recover from these disabilities, but the fact that he would fly into sudden rages did disconcert him. He pressed his wife and the doctors to tell him what was the matter; however, even though they attempted to explain it to him, he simply would not listen. Long afterward he recognized that he was using the defense of intellectual denial.

He wrote: "I heeded only the most optimistic things that were said to me and the rest, I did not hear them or came to the conclusion that they were wrong" (p. 22). As a result he was very critical of the doctors and nurses — it simply confirmed that "all doctors are imbeciles." He felt that once he learned the secret ("when the switch is turned on"), then his tongue would be loosened. In the meantime, since he was unable to speak, his wife and he adapted the game of Twenty Questions to meet his needs.

At home the long, difficult job of recovery now faced Ritchie, and he sought out various therapists other than doctors; a physiotherapist took charge. Ritchie felt confidence in the therapist and eventually he began to walk again.

He also began speech therapy, but so disliked the therapist ("she treated me like a small child") that eventually he discontinued treatment. Ten months after the stroke he was accepted at a medical rehabilitiation center, and from that point much of his time was spent in physiologic therapy, occupational therapy, and speech therapy. He could not detect any improvement in his speech and finally abandoned speech lessons again, although he was still confident that he would learn to speak normally (he was still searching for the "switch"). Ritchie disliked the other patients at the center intensely. Many of them were stroke patients similar to himself.

Three months later he slipped away from the center, thinking that he would not have to return, but while on vacation he was confronted with his forced retirement from BBC. His morale hit rock bottom, and thoughts of suicide filled his mind, so he returned to the rehabilitation center. He observed that it was one thing to think and quite another to put thoughts into words. "I could think, actively, without using words, and coming down to earth, I rehearsed speeches silently. But there was the blank wall. The minute I rehearsed speeches with my tongue, even though I kept silent, the words would not come" (p. 56).

In the second year, despair slowly gave rise to hope. He became friendly with an extroverted war veteran at the center. He also entered speech therapy again and this time found that he liked his new therapist. Most important of all, he stated that "Underneath, I had a new kind of confidence. Not confidence in doctors, in instructors, in physiotherapists, in speech therapists, that they could command health to return to my body. I had nearly rid myself of the idea of them as witch doctors. Dating from the summer before, when my morale hit bottom, I had confidence in nobody but myself" (p. 87). It took two years before he worked through the defense of insulation and decided that his recovery depended largely on himself. He lamented the lost time, but settled down to work hard on his remaining symptoms. (However, one can see the function that his defense had served — it saved him from depression and possible suicide.)

Twenty-two months after the stroke he hit on the idea of writing about his experience. In May his senses of taste and smell came back; in July he wrote that "My speech is definitely better and my writing much improved" (he had thought that writing was related to reading, but found it was much closer to speech); and in August he dreamed for the first time since the stroke. He was discharged from the center in December. A month later he wrote a cryptic note that the director of the center had died of a cerebral hemorrhage.

His speech therapist with whom he continued tried to get him to give up writing the account of his stroke, but he persisted. Even though the memory of his past ills seemed to cause psychosomatic ailments, he felt compelled to complete the account. A brief chapter written ten years later stated that he was then able to walk a half-mile per day with a leg iron; his right arm was still useless (apparently only one in ten stroke victims recovers useful function of the arm); his speech was reportedly 40 to 60 percent of normal, but he felt that it was still improving; and his comprehension was 80 to 90 percent of normal. The last line stated that "Life immediately after the stroke was simply incomprehensible, now it is full of surprises, excitement and satisfaction."

The second author was Eric Hodgins, a writer and a journalist. He had written several books, the best known being *Mr. Blanding Builds His Dream House.* Hodgins was sixty when the "episode" took place. The book about the "accident inside his skull" (1964) is worth mentioning for several reasons: (1) the author did recover a considerable amount of his literary skill in a relatively short period of time, which leads to the conjecture about the severity of the stroke or the fact that having a sizable literary skill may somehow compensate for brain damage; (2) his recovery was largely spontaneous rather than due to any professional help that he received; and (3) he was divorced and had to recover without assistance from any members of his family.

Hodgins was paralyzed on the left side and at first was aphasic, as a great number of people are immediately after they receive a stroke. His mind was also confused, but in a day or so his mind cleared up. The treatment in the hospital was physiotherapy only; nothing was done about his speech, but it slowly came back by itself. He was also plagued by a faulty memory. In terms of background he indicates a history of high blood pressure and a chronic heart condition.

In about four weeks he left the hospital and returned home. He disliked his night nurse because she was so "goody-goody" and staunchily religious; he liked his day nurse better and admits to having his "first carnal thoughts" about her. He began speech therapy, but the therapist concluded that his speech would return without formal speech training. This was fine with Hodgins since he didn't like the therapist either. But he did like his physical therapist, and rapid progress was made in getting him to walk again.

Seven months after the accident, he entered a psychiatric resident clinic because he was a definite suicidal risk. He was treated with recreational therapy, occupational therapy, sedation, and psychotherapy. In his book he never did describe what the content of psychotherapy was all about except to deride generally the treatment he received. He spent three months in the clinic and, despite his expressed doubts, left without the suicidal impulses.

Eighteen months after discharge from the clinic he fell, cracking his right hip, and ended up in the hospital again. He again was very derogatory about the treatment that he received, but he did state that one way the fall had worked to his advantage was that he got to use a cane, which signaled to others that he had some affliction. His improvement continued and at the conclusion of the book he was writing with a ballpoint pen held in the right hand (he never learned to use the typewriter again). In an appendix he pointed out that medical treatment cost over $22,000 in eighteen months. There is one other point worth emphasizing in Hodgins's case. The thrombosis settled in his right hemisphere but his admitted transferred right-handedness at an early age (he probably did not have a dominant hemisphere) could have salvaged much of his influency.

The third book, *Pat and Roald,* concerned the actress Patricia Neal, and was written by a professional journalist (Farrell, 1969). It detailed what happened to Pat from the time of her stroke in February, 1965, through a period of intensive rehabilitation in 1968. It is my firm impression that Patricia Neal may have been the only person reported in the literature to respond to a definite remedial program which was laid down by someone else.

Pat was thirty-nine when she sustained three gross hemorrhages in an hour or two, the third while she was on the operating table for repair of the effects of the first two. Very fortunately, her husband, Roald Dahl, knew a lot about neurophysiological processes, because of an accident undergone by one of their children, and he happened to have the phone number of a famous neurosurgeon at the UCLA medical school. As it was, Pat was in a coma for fourteen days and was silent for a week longer before she uttered her first sound.

Subsequently Dahl was a tremendous, vigorous force in getting Pat well. He hounded, cajoled, and wheedled her. It seems he simply had his mind made up that a full recovery was possible without hedges or conditions. As everyone knows, the first six months following a stroke are accepted as the period of greatest spontaneous recovery, and in a sense this was true of Pat. Upon leaving the hospital her eyesight was impaired (she suffered double vision), her right arm and leg were useless, she was aphasic, her memory was such that she couldn't even remember her husband's or her children's names, and her concentration was very poor. After six months, Dahl judged that her recovery was 60 percent complete. But in another sense she was just beginning the process of becoming Pat Neal again.

Adding to the complications was Pat's pregnancy — she was in the fourth month and gave birth to a normal girl five months later. The birth of the baby reportedly gave her a great boost of morale. The technique that Dahl used for rehabilitation is interesting. He gathered the neighbors around Pat and assigned many of the volunteers jobs as therapists; at first extremely hesitant to accept this responsibility, they quickly developed into very competent teachers. Dahl reserved his strength for running the house and family, and for earning a living as a writer. He got others to do the actual retraining and teaching. Readers might be interested in his specific program, which is laid down on pages 147-152 in the book.

While some people may react against Dahl's dictatorial pressure in getting Pat to work so extraordinarily diligently, be under no illusion that remediation from such a severe stroke calls for anything but adherence to the most compulsive program. Two years after the stroke, Pat traveled to Washington to receive the "Heart of the Year" award from President Johnson. Early in 1968 she acted in *The Subject Was Roses,* a movie performance for which she received an Oscar nomination.

The paramount feature of the book seems to be that under prolonged and expert guidance, a stroke victim can be helped. To me it showed a combination of the advantages of luck (that the stroke didn't totally disable her), of an immensely intelligent and stubborn husband (one who could sustain a high level of morale and still keep her constantly driving), of a lot of friends (who were marshaled about her as teachers), and of ample money (although it was not stressed, her treatment did cost a great deal).

The next to last book was one written by Buck (1968) expressly for speech therapists and other professional workers who are confronted with the treatment of aphasics, or rather dysphasics (a dysphasic suffers from a slight or moderate neurological difficulty, still has a store of language relatively intact, and is educable or trainable; the aphasic is one who has suffered much greater brain damage and whose recovery is much more difficult or even impossible). Buck labels himself as a dysphasic. The main thesis of his book is that a stroke is a family illness and professional assistance should be readily available for the entire household, which of course reflects what Buck found to be valuable in his rehabilitation. It is of interest that Buck's professional friends and colleagues were distraught over his complete rejection of their commercial language drills, machines, and books.

Rather than concentrate on the book per se, which I have heard discussed by speech therapists pro and con, let me comment on Buck's personal article in which he details the stroke that befell him in 1957, which was six years before the article and twelve years before he got around to writing the book. Let me focus on just one important insight. Near the end of the two-page article he delivers a rather profound statement, one which I do not remember reading elsewhere (perhaps it could be inferred from his book, but it was less obviously stated). Buck says that he found no assistance whatsoever from direct vocabulary and language drills — the majority of his successes were almost wholly dependent upon his psychological security and the deletion of unrealistic pressures concerning word-by-word expression in conversation.

To put it another way, only when Buck was able to ignore his listeners and concentrate upon his thought processes did he begin to demonstrate progress in free expression. The less he concentrated upon individual words, the more meaningful his expression became. In other words, he attempted to feel as natural or normal as those about him and to act accordingly by not paying undue attention to word selection, although this required an abundance of self-discipline. The attempt was to get back to the normal "unconscious" sort of speaking where the machinery goes on more or less automatically. According to Buck, he attempted to feel as normal as other people do, or as he did before he encountered the stroke. This to my mind is exactly the opposite of what most patients and the majority of speech therapists attempt to do.

In conclusion, Buck cautions that he still suffers from unpredictable periods of difficulty concerning the recall of proper names, and he has no explanation of these apparent neurological short circuits.[2] But nothing impresses like success — he eventually took a position as the head of speech pathology at a medical school.

Behavioral Changes Following Strokes (Ullman, 1962) differs from the foregoing highly selected and admittedly biased articles and books. The principal investigator reports on his experiences in seeing 300 stroke patients during a three-year period. Excerpts were taken from sixty-four of these cases; all of the patients were from the lower socioeconomic level. There were partial remissions over time — people did get well enough to go home and a few of these even got well enough to go back to work — though the study did not follow the patients over an extended period of time. No patient studied under this research grant demonstrated anything near the remarkable recovery manifested in the previous articles.

So what are my tentative conclusions?

1. From my immersion into the self-reports of aphasics, which after all are only a few single reports without any control whatsoever, I am nevertheless left with the probable belief that now and then something can speed their partial recovery. However, I am also convinced that neurologically traumatized individuals seldom return to their pre-traumatic levels of functioning. Even the most recovered person is left with the lingering, nagging doubt, "Will I be able to verbalize the next word or sentence or keep the concept in mind while we discuss it?"

2. It seems that there has been no real breakthrough in retraining procedures — nothing in the way of any standardized treatment techniques exist. The majority of aphasics go to speech therapists who frankly do not know how to assist them with more than the most fundamental rehabilitation. But on the other hand, no therapist, be he physician, speech therapist, or psychologist, knows much about the inner world of the aphasic or what can be done to remedy it.

[2] This is apparently again difficulty in rote memory.

3. The main quality of the uniquely individualized remediation seems to be the sustained high level of motivation on the part of the aphasic, which builds upon "spontaneous recovery." It is strictly trial and error when the patient happens to hit on something that seems effective for him. On the other hand, I am convinced that retraining can go on longer than one month or even six months.

4. Since the stroke, like any other form of natural catastrophe, is greatly debilitating and no type of treatment is effective at the present time, it does seem that some kind of national health insurance could be of financial aid to the disabled worker.

5. We are at the stage where careful, systematic, highly imaginative research must play the most significant role. Unfortunately, we are still at the pilot or exploratory level.

References

Albertson, E. T. 1947. A glimpse into an aphasic's world. *American Journal of Occupational Therapy,* 1, 361-64.

Buck, M. 1963. The language disorders: a personal and professional account of aphasia. *Journal of Rehabilitation,* 29, 37-38.

———. 1968. *Dysphasia: professional guidance from family and patients,* Englewood Cliffs, N. J.: Prentice-Hall.

Critchley, M. 1962. Dr. Samuel Johnson's aphasia. *Medical History,* 6, 27-46.

Farrell, B. 1969. *Pat and Roald.* New York: Random House.

Hall, W. A. 1961. Return from silence: a personal experience, *Journal of Speech and Hearing Disorders,* 26, 174-76.

Hodgins, E. 1964. *Episode: report on the accident inside my skull.* New York: Atheneum.

Hoff, H. E., Guillemin, R., and Geddes, L. A. 1958. An 18th century scientist's observations of his own aphasia. *Bulletin of Historical Medicine,* 32, 446-50.

Osthoff, F. I. 1970. Accurate empathy in helping professional trainees as related to reading experiences. Unpublished Ph.D. dissertation, Univerity of Illinois.

Riese, W. 1954. Auto-observation reported by eminent nineteenth century medical scientist. *Bulletin of Historical Medicine,* 28, 237-42.

Ritchie, D. 1966. *Stroke: a diary of recovery.* London: Faber and Faber.

Rolnick, M., and Hoops, H. R. 1970. Aphasia as seen by the aphasic. *Journal of Speech and Hearing Disorders,* 34, 48-53.

Rose, R. H. 1948. A physician's account of his own aphasia. *Journal of Speech and Hearing Disorders,* 13, 294-305.

Sies, L. F., and Butler, B. 1963. A personal account of dysphasia, *Journal of Speech and Hearing Disorders,* 28, 261-66.

Ullman, M. 1962. *Behavioral changes in patients following strokes,* Springfield, Ill.: C. C. Thomas.

Index